KU-084-653

The Body Control

Pilates Pregnancy Book

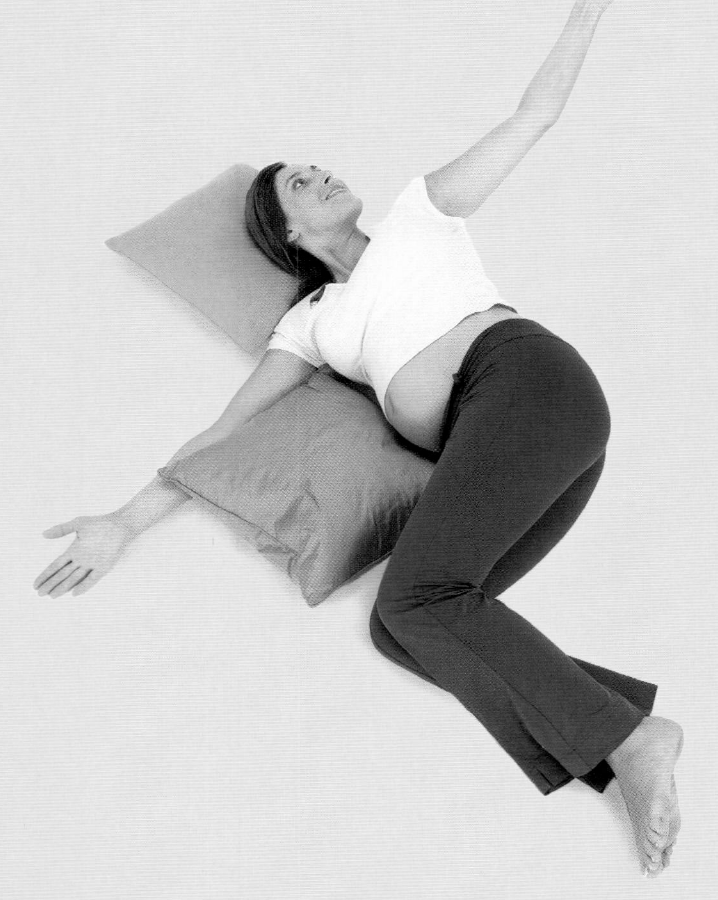

LYNNE ROBINSON
Medical Consultant JACQUELINE KNOX MCSP SRP

The Body Control

Pilates Pregnancy Book

Optimum Health and Fitness for Every Stage of Your Pregnancy

Pan Books

First published 2004 by Pan Books
an imprint of Pan Macmillan Ltd
Pan Macmillan, 20 New Wharf Road, London N1 9RR
Basingstoke and Oxford
Associated companies throughout the world
www.panmacmillan.com

ISBN 0 330 41235 3

9 8 7 6 5 4 3 2 1

A CIP catalogue record for this book is available from the British Library.

Typeset by SX Composing DTP, Rayleigh, Essex
Colour Reproduction by Aylesbury Studios (Bromley) Ltd
Printed and bound in Great Britain by Butler and Tanner, Frome, Somerset.

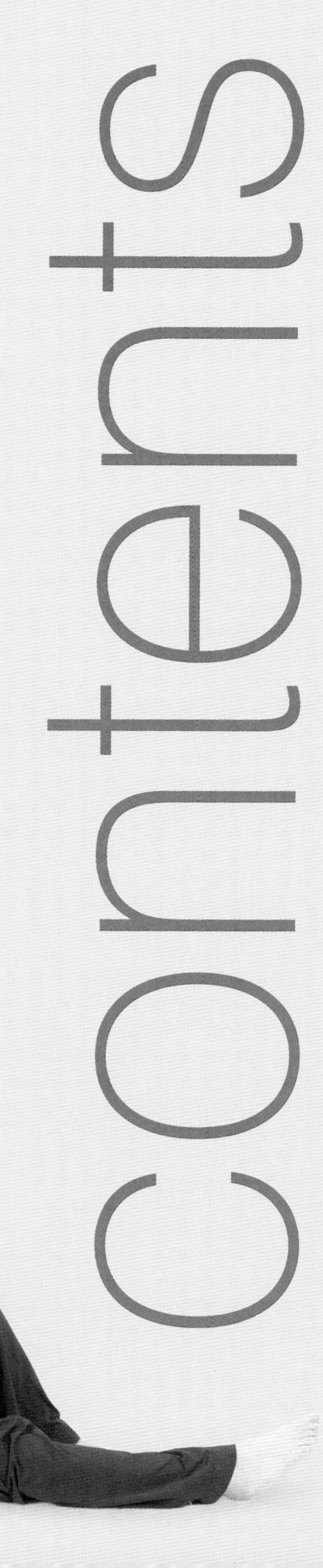
contents

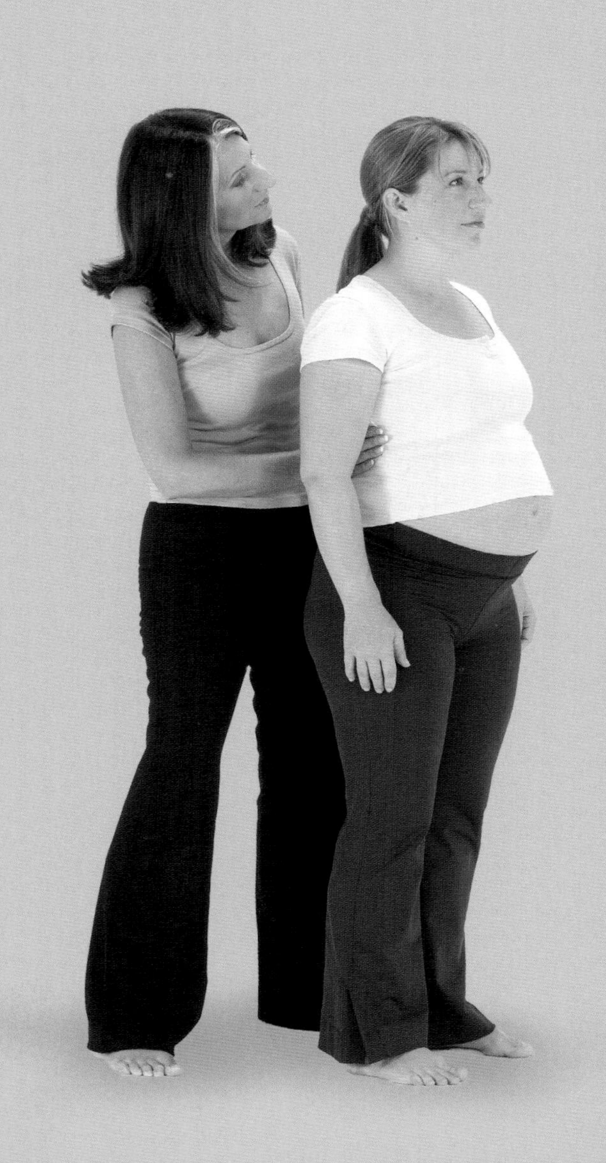

1 The Benefits of Pilates During Pregnancy

Women today enter into pregnancy and labour well informed about tests, foods and so on, but often forget the most important factor: fitness. Women are often physically unfit for pregnancy and labour. – Lisa Marshall, Midwife

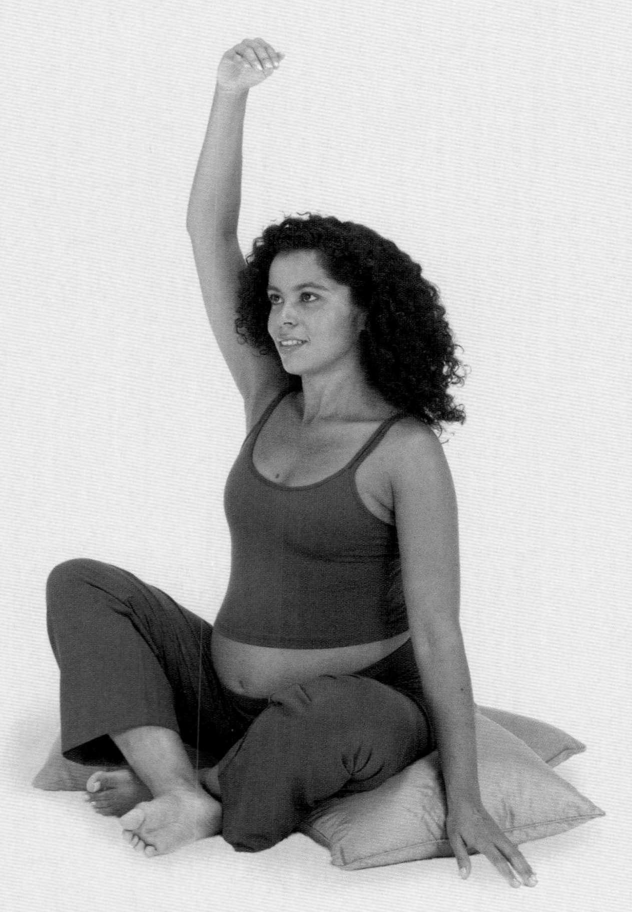

If you have chosen to read this book the chances are that you are either pregnant, planning to have a baby or are a health professional with a specialist interest in antenatal and post-natal women. Whichever is the case, you recognize the importance of keeping fit and healthy during pregnancy. As more and more fitness centres open, we are faced with an array of different exercise classes ranging from mind–body techniques such as yoga, Pilates and tai-chi to purely physical activities such as step aerobics, core training, body pump and combat and, of course, the familiar gym machines. If you already exercise regularly, you will be wondering if you can continue with your normal class while pregnant. Is it safe?

When you are pregnant your exercise priorities change. Pregnancy is a perfectly normal state – you are not ill – but as a pregnant woman your exercise needs will change month by month. In the chapters that follow, we will look at the way in which your body alters, and why you need to adapt your exercise routine. Body Control Pilates is the safest, most effective and, hopefully, the most enjoyable exercise method you can do at this very exciting time.

Why Is Pilates so Perfect for Pregnancy?

Pregnancy is a time when you undergo enormous emotional, physical and hormonal changes. Any exercise you decide to do must take these changes into account. Now is not the time to attempt to get super fit, super toned or, indeed, super slim! Your priority is to maintain a level of fitness that is beneficial to you and to your baby.

What you need is an exercise method that prepares you for the rigours of labour which is what it says it is – extremely hard work – and for motherhood! You need a method that:

- ensures your body's systems – circulatory, lymphatic, respiratory, digestive – are all functioning efficiently, so that you and your growing baby are healthy
- helps make your pregnancy comfortable and pain free
- teaches you to relax, which will be invaluable throughout your pregnancy, during the birth itself and as you care for your newborn baby
- gives you both the opportunity and tools you need to get to know your body and be aware of its needs
- prepares you for labour
- And last, but by no means least, you need a method that lays the foundations to help you get your figure back after the birth.

The Body Control Pilates Method can meet all these needs and more. Pilates is essentially a mind and body training method. You learn to move correctly, thoughtfully and mindfully. The slow, controlled movements of the exercises are non-impact, and so will not stress your joints, and are very safe for the pregnant mother. Pilates, with its emphasis on correct alignment and good posture, is perfect because pregnancy is a time when your posture can change quite dramatically. Let's look at the upper body – as your breasts grow and become heavier there is an increased strain on your neck, shoulders and upper back. Pilates teaches you how to release tension, improve your awareness of good upper-body movement and strengthen the mid-back muscles, which prevent you from becoming round shouldered. At the same time, the exercises help prepare your upper body for the demands of breast feeding and infant care.

Pilates is an excellent way to strengthen postural muscles through increased body awareness. This is so valuable during pregnancy when associated changes in the body can lead to numerous aches and pains. Practising Pilates through pregancy will not only help to train the muscles which support and protect against such problems but will also develop skills useful during labour, and help to prepare for the demands of motherhood.

– Philippa Satchwell, Physiotherapist

Your Natural Girdle of Strength

Where Pilates is unique is in its focus on the deep postural muscles of the body, on your 'core muscles'. In particular, Pilates strengthens your transversus abdominis muscle which wraps itself around your torso like a natural corset. As your uterus grows, this 'girdle of strength' will support your bump and also protect your spine. In the course of a single hour of Pilates, you do hundreds of abdominal exercises, because every time you move, you engage this deep transversus muscle in an action we call 'zip up and hollow'. It is also worth noting that transversus is also a key muscle used during labour itself – it is the muscle you use to push!

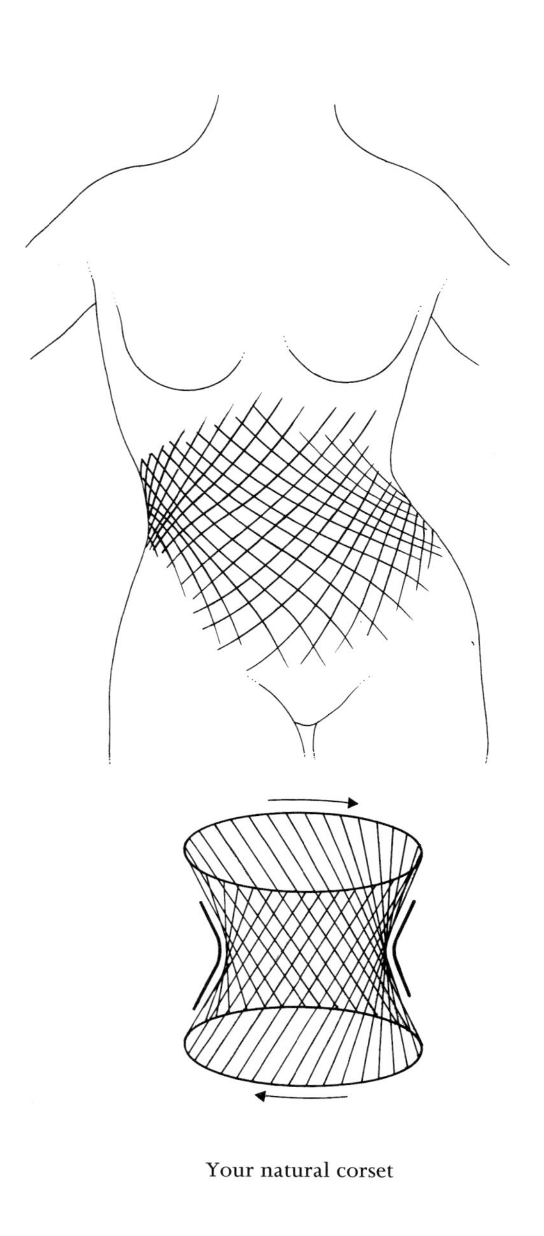

Your natural corset

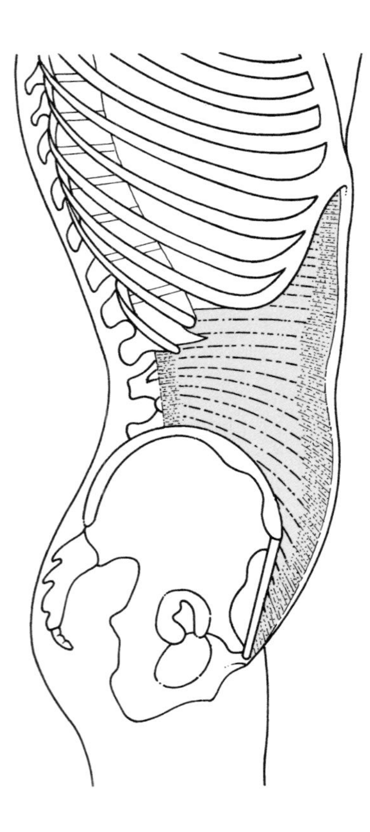

Transversus abdominis

In order to allow the uterus to grow, the superficial abdominal muscle, the rectus abdominis (commonly called the six-pack muscle) separates in what is called diastasis recti. Once this happens in the second trimester the traditional curl-up exercises are no longer recommended (see page 117). Many pregnant mothers despair that they will ever regain a flat stomach after the birth unless they work this six-pack muscle, and there is a great temptation to do these exercises which can in fact lead to the abdominals being strengthened apart! The rectus abdominis is not nearly as important as you think in achieving good abdominal tone. Notice from the diagram that the fibres of the rectus abdominis run from top to bottom. Now, think of an old-fashioned corset – in which direction do the fibres of the corset run? They run horizontally, criss-crossing and wrapping around the trunk. If you are anxious about regaining your shape, then focus on your transversus abdominis (using the zip up and hollow) and the obliques by doing Hip Rolls (page 81) for example.

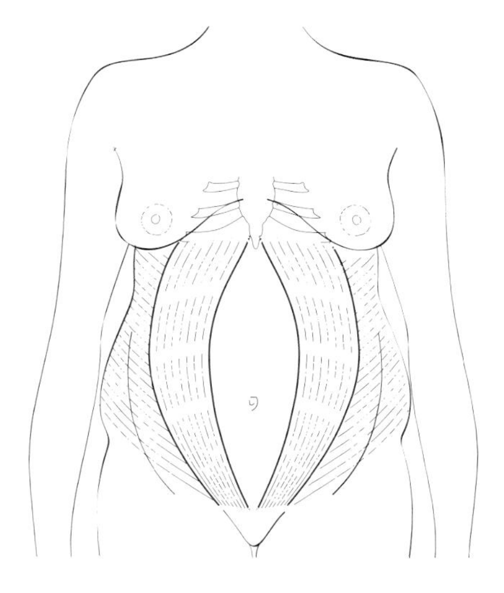

Diastasis recti – the rectus separates

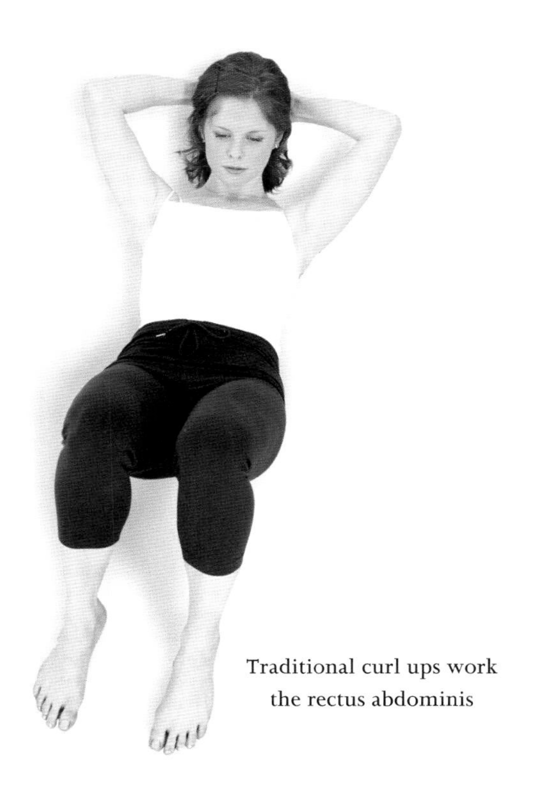

Traditional curl ups work the rectus abdominis

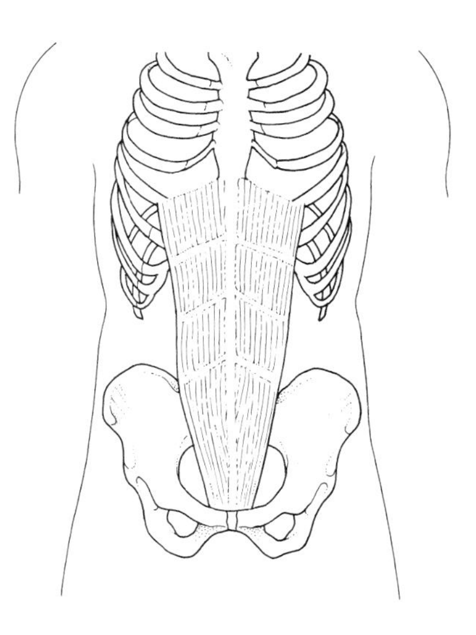

Rectus abdominis (six-pack)

Working the Pelvic Floor

Even more exciting is that in Pilates you not only work on the abdominals, you also simultaneously work the pelvic floor, that's the 'zip' part of the action. By the time you begin labour, you will be very familiar with your pelvic floor. Some mothers worry that strong pelvic floor muscles will result in a difficult birth, but by doing Pilates you will learn how to control those muscles. They will be strong, but you will also have learnt how to release them for the final stages of delivery. Good pelvic floor muscles will help prevent incontinence and improve your sex life. Pelvic floor exercises will also improve circulation to the pelvic area, help improve the functioning of the reproductive organs and aid the healing process after the birth itself.

As the uterus becomes heavier, it is the pelvic floor that must bear the weight. It may drop as much as 2.5 centimetres (1 inch), not to mention the fact that towards the end of your pregnancy the baby is likely to use the pelvic floor just like a trampoline!

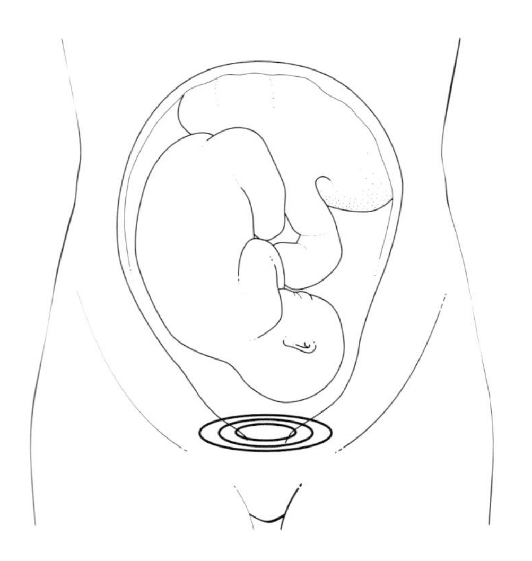

The pelvic floor bears the weight of the uterus and the baby

If we haven't convinced you yet of the importance of the pelvic floor then perhaps the following illustration will help: if you had to carry a cardboard box full of heavy bottles, how would you carry it? Would you just hold the sides of the box? Of course not, you would support it from underneath.

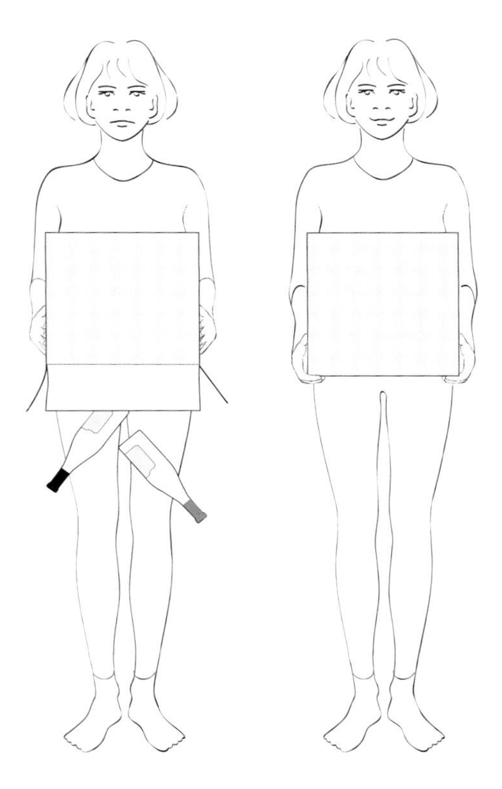

Using the pelvic floor gives you maximum support

Hormonal Change and Joint Instability

When you are pregnant, your body is on a hormone roller coaster and has 100 per cent more progesterone and oestrogen. These hormones soften the muscles, allowing the baby to grow. Meanwhile, an increase in the hormone relaxin affects the collagen in the ligaments. Ligaments join bone to bone and help provide stability at a joint. Normally they are non-elastic, like cotton or linen, but during pregnancy they lose a lot of tensile strength and become more elastic, like lycra. This allows the pelvis to widen in preparation for the birth. As a result, all your joints become more mobile, and you, in fact, become more supple. This sounds like a good thing, but the problem is that your joints also become less stable. Many pregnant women develop joint problems for the first time during pregnancy. Sacroiliac joint problems (where the sacrum joins the pelvis) are common.

To see why, let's look at the pelvis. Basically your pelvis normally gets its stability from what is referred to as 'form closure' and 'force closure'. Form closure is the natural stability you get from your anatomy, from the structure of the joints and their opposing surfaces. The sacrum sits firmly like a wedge in between the two ilia in the pelvis, with strong ligaments holding the bones in place. Force closure is the extra stability you get from external forces to keep the joints in place. This is not to do with the shape of the pelvis, but with the force applied from the outside – that is, from your muscles.

We have already seen that during pregnancy your ligaments soften and become like lycra, which effectively results in a loss of stability in the pelvis: you lose your form closure. This is when your stabilizing muscles, therefore, become very important. Stabilizing muscles are sometimes called fixating muscles in that they hold your bones in good alignment allowing free movement around a joint. Pilates, with its focus on good alignment and proper muscle recruitment, strengthens these deep core muscles and thus helps to prevent the sacroiliac and pubic joint problems that often occur in pregnancy.

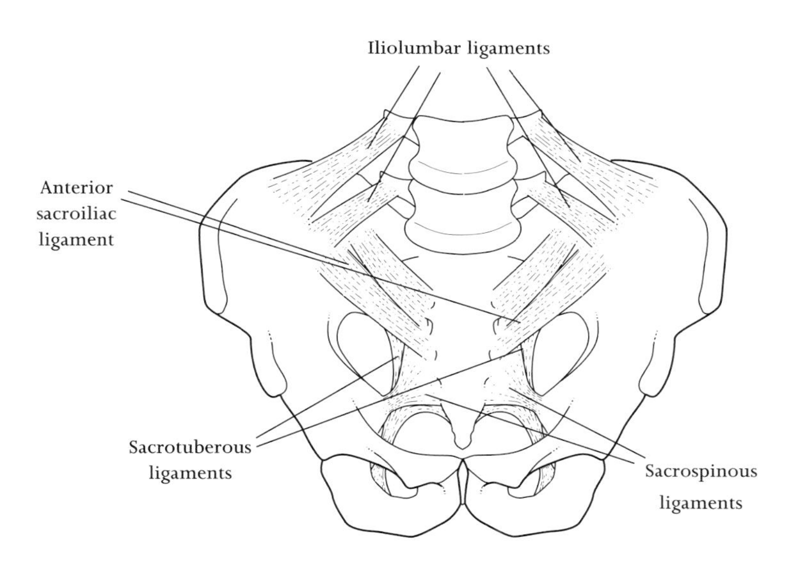

Strong ligaments hold the pelvic bones in place

Fluid Retention and Circulation Problems

During pregnancy, your blood volume is going to increase by as much as 40 per cent. This, not surprisingly, puts extra pressure on the heart, which has to pump it around your body. Your heart is the most important muscle in your body and it needs to be able to cope with this extra demand. Hopefully, you will have included some kind of aerobic exercise in your fitness regime before you became pregnant. You should continue with gentle cardiovascular work through your pregnancy, but you should be careful not to raise your heart rate or your body temperature too high (see page 40). The exercises in this book will not dramatically raise your heart rate, but they should ensure that your movements are pain free, and they work on improving your circulation.

Veins carry blood from the extremities back to the heart. To do this they have to work against gravity. To help them, they have a series of valves that prevent the back flow of blood. Unfortunately, hormonal changes can affect the working of the valves, and blood can pool in the veins, especially in the legs and the rectum. This results in a bulging of the veins and causes varicose veins and haemorrhoids. The extra weight gain in pregnancy, the relaxation of the muscle tissue, the increase in blood volume and the added pressure of the uterus on the pelvic area all compound the problem. Fortunately, there are lots of Pilates exercises which work the deep calf pumps, boosting the circulation in the lower limbs.

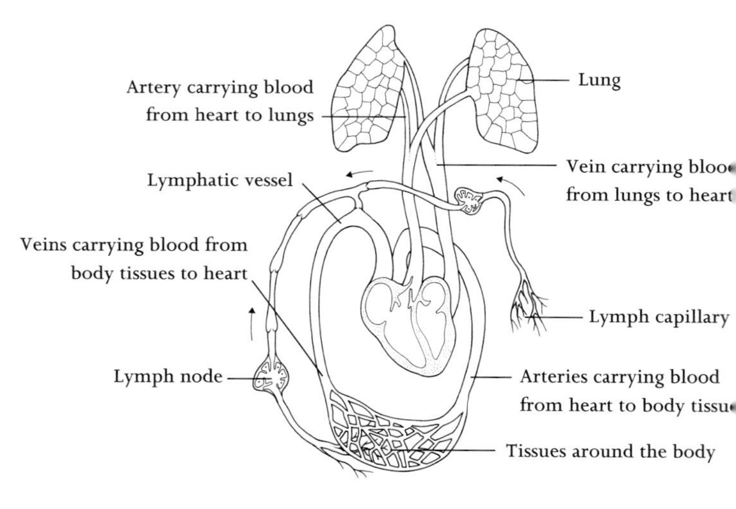

Lymphatic system

As a heavy rainstorm freshens the water of a stagnant stream and whips it into immediate action, so does the Pilates Method purify the blood stream. – Joseph Pilates

In addition to the increase in blood volume there is also an increase in fluid to all the body's tissues, including lymphatic fluid which, essentially, is the body's waste-disposal system. As a result, fluid retention can become a problem. Pregnant women may suffer from oedema, a mild swelling of the ankles and feet. Once again, many Pilates exercises help to improve lymphatic drainage, which relies on muscular action in the legs, and thus help to keep those fluids moving.

Breathing and Relaxation

Correct breathing is an essential part of the Pilates method, it is one of the basic Eight Principles (page 28). Pilates uses lateral thoracic breathing, which involves breathing into the sides and back of the ribcage. One of the things you learn is how to exhale fully, 'wringing out the lungs'. When you do this you get rid of non-beneficial gases and other toxins. And the more you can wring out your lungs, the better able you are to draw in the oxygen you need to reach your muscles and help you relax. In the later trimesters, as your baby grows, your ribcage will elevate and you may find yourself increasingly short of breath. Pilates breathing will help increase your lung capacity and help you cope with this shortness of breath.

Learning how to release tension in the body is a starting point for Pilates. It is our very first principle. After doing a Pilates session the level of the stress hormone cortisol drops significantly – leaving you feeling calm and stress free. Getting adequate rest throughout your pregnancy is as important as getting adequate exercise. It can help with hypertension (high blood pressure), back problems, indigestion and even, looking ahead, breastfeeding. You will feel better equipped to manage stress and you are providing all the positive health benefits of a stress-free environment for yourself and your baby (and your partner!).

But it is during labour that the ability to relax becomes vital. Pilates gives you an awareness of the breath; it teaches you to use the breath to release tension, to control movement and to breathe through discomfort. Once learnt, these tools will prove invaluable, not only during your pregnancy, but during labour itself.

Pilates relaxation is of great benefit in labour, helping women to focus on the work the body is doing. The breathing and relaxation will help the journey through labour to safe delivery of the baby. – Lisa Marshall, Midwife

. . . To breathe correctly you must completely exhale and inhale, always trying very hard to squeeze every atom of impure air from your lungs in much the same manner that you would wring every drop of water from a wet cloth . . . the lungs will automatically completely refill themselves with fresh air. This in turn supplies the bloodstream with vitally necessary life-giving oxygen. – Joseph Pilates

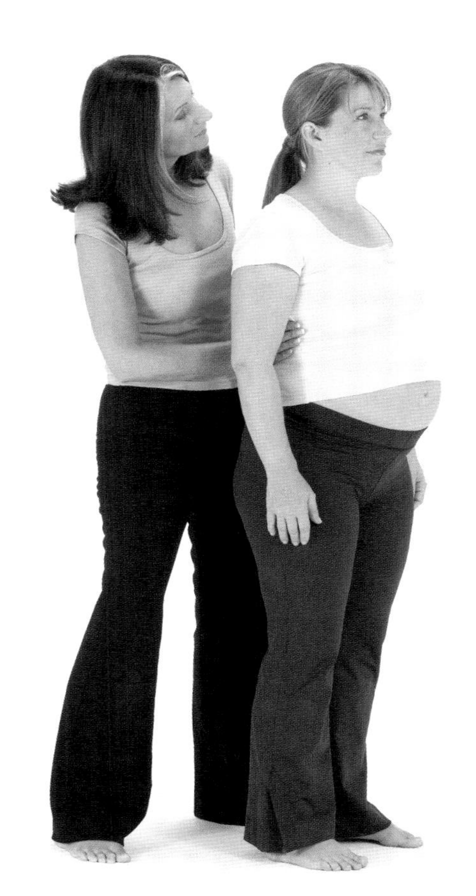

Feeling Good

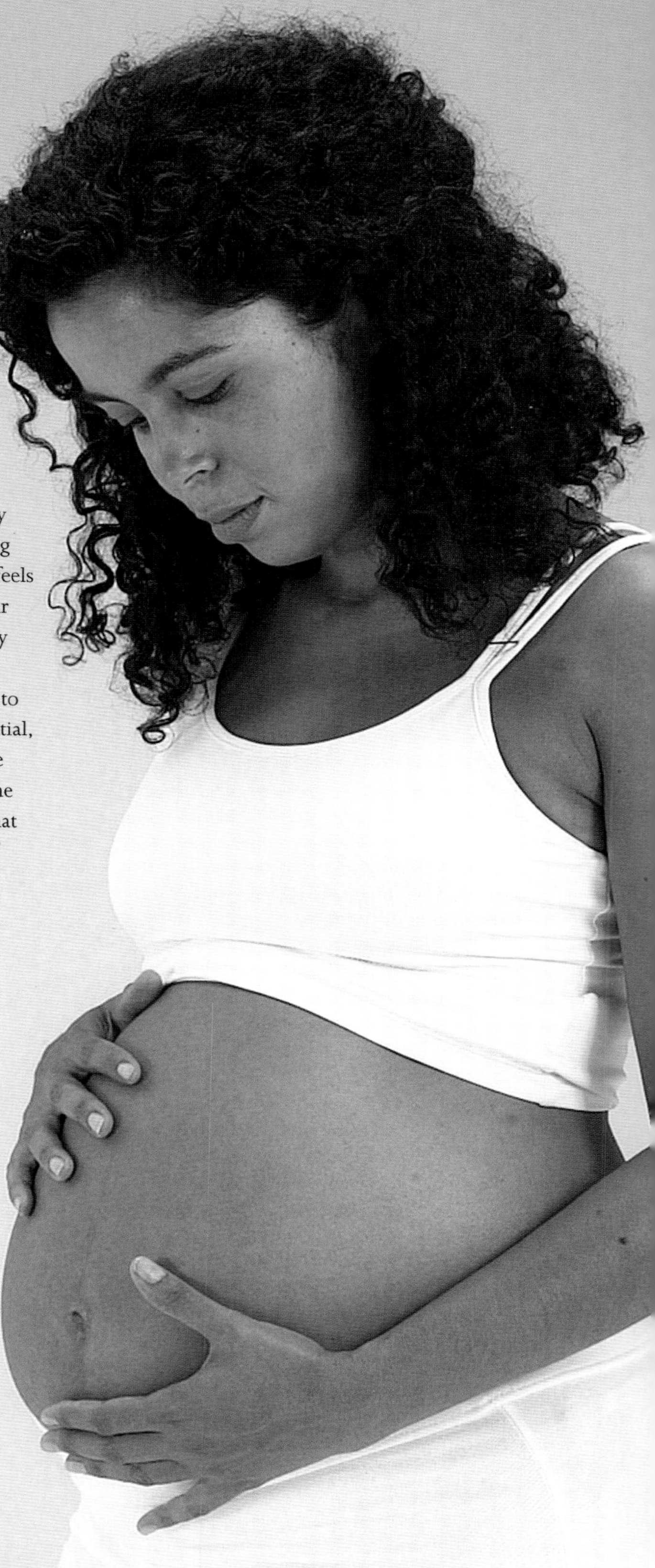

Finally, we should not underestimate the psychological benefits of exercising throughout your pregnancy. Carrying a child is one of the most profound and magical things a woman can do, but as thrilling as it is, it is also a daunting experience. Sometimes you can feel as though you have lost control of your body. This can be bewildering especially for a first-time mother. Pilates can help to give you that control back. As your body awareness improves, as your body strengthens, you feel as though you are back in the driving seat.

The feel-good endorphins that are released naturally after any type of exercise play a valuable role in keeping your spirits high and in giving you self-confidence. It feels good to keep active. You may not be able to touch your toes or even see them, but you can still move gracefully and freely while performing your exercises.

Use your Pilates sessions as quality 'me time', time to reflect, and find inner calm and harmony. This is essential, particularly if you have other children to look after, are working and/or have very little time for yourself. At the end of the day, you can relax, safe in the knowledge that you have chosen the best possible exercise for yourself and your baby.

The Importance of Good Posture

When you are pregnant, the increased weight gain, most of which is carried in front, is clearly going to affect your posture. Women who normally have excellent posture often find that it deteriorates during their pregnancy. In fact, your whole balance and centre of gravity changes: it no longer falls over the feet. You may feel the need to lean back to correct this shift in the centre of gravity, but not every woman responds the same way. The traditional 'pregnancy stance' seen below is common, but posture is very individual and you should try to maintain your normal spinal alignment.

Before we look at what happens to your posture while pregnant, let's look at normal posture. If you look up the word posture in a dictionary you will find the following definitions:

- a particular position of the body
- a characteristic or assumed bearing, specifically the pose of a model or a figure
- an attitude
- a state or frame of mind

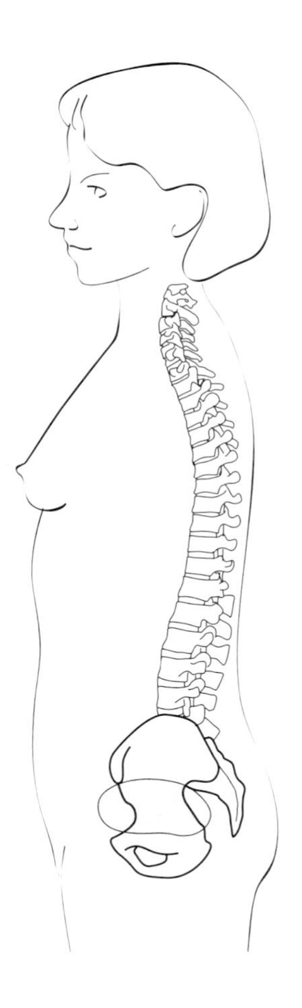

Non-pregnant posture

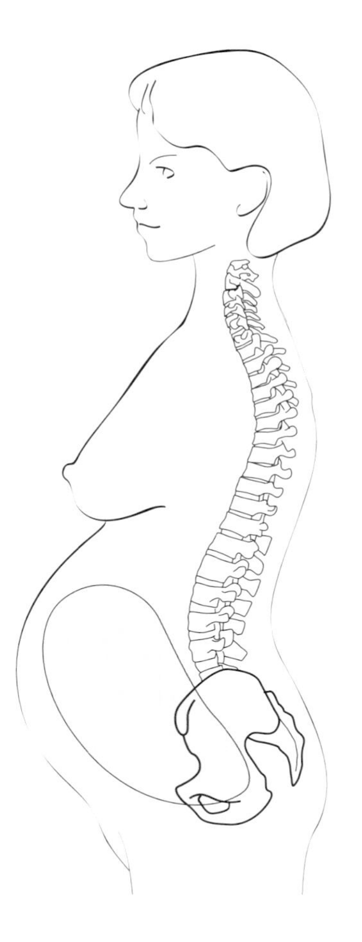

Typical pregnant posture

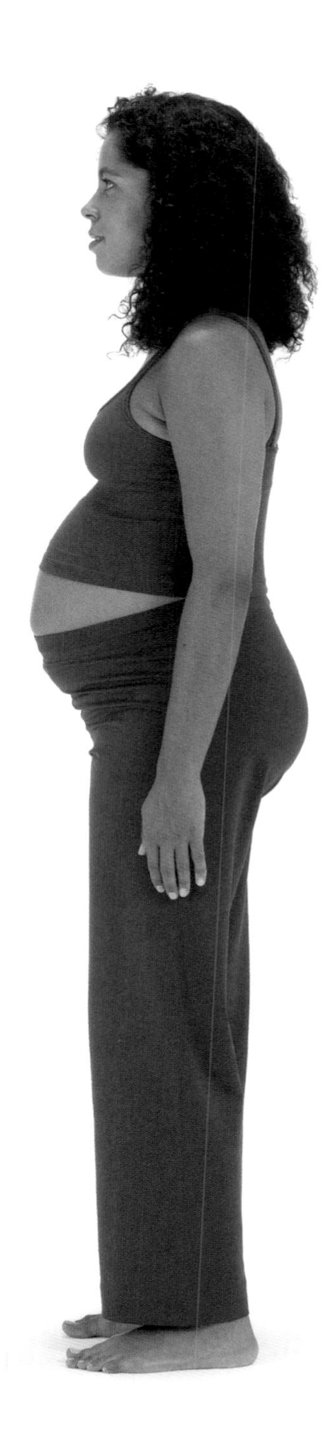

Did the last two definitions surprise you? They shouldn't, because your posture is a clear giveaway of how you are feeling, what you think about yourself, and how you want the world to see you. Over the next few paragraphs, we are going to give you very definite guidelines of what we believe good posture to be – of the correct alignment of bones, the correct recruitment of muscles. But we need to remember that posture is dynamic, it is freedom of movement, an expression of self-awareness. You cannot 'hold' good posture – pulling your shoulders back, squeezing your buttocks, standing straight, holding your stomach in – this only serves to create tension, which ultimately restricts freedom of movement. If you want to improve your posture you need to become body aware, and bring a new level of awareness to everything you do – not just to your exercises. For that, we have to change something that is subconscious, that is automatic.

Movement and the control of movement originate in the nervous system. When we were young we learnt to reach, sit, crawl, stand and walk, by watching, imitating, trying, making mistakes, and then learning from those mistakes. We tried and tried again until we got it right, until the action was ingrained. Once a movement is ingrained or grooved, it becomes automatic – a muscle memory. If we are going to re-learn how to stand, sit and move, we have to start at the beginning again. To watch, learn and then practise again and again until that movement, that way of standing, sitting or moving is ingrained and automatic. This is where Pilates comes into its own because, with each exercise, you are taken through a good movement pattern. These patterns are repeated continually in different exercises, until the movements are ingrained in our subconscious.

Good posture and movement are at the heart of the Pilates Method. Clients at Joseph Pilates' New York studio were reprimanded for sitting or standing badly (sometimes quite harshly!). As they learned his exercises and worked on his studio machines, they not only became stronger and more flexible but they also re-learned how to move. This doesn't happen overnight; it is a slow process. But the exercises and instructions given in this book will ultimately change your posture and the way you move. Gradually you wake up to being body aware. This is why we strongly recommend that you start Pilates before you become pregnant.

We know that during pregnancy your body is going to be changing daily: the centre of gravity changes, posture changes. It is much easier to adapt to these changes if you already have good body awareness and posture.

The benefits of good posture should not be underestimated. It may help you avoid the aches and pains associated with back and joint problems throughout the body. It will help you look great. Nothing is as unflattering as poor posture – it can make you look shorter, make your breasts look saggy, your waist thicker, your stomach and your bottom bigger.

In ideal posture the forces of gravity are evenly distributed through the body. All joints are in their neutral zone. There will be minimal wear and tear on these structures and the natural balance and correct length of the muscles is maintained. The muscles are balanced and therefore movement patterns are normal. All the vital organs are properly placed and not constricted, so they function better.

Notice the points of the body through which the imaginary plumbline falls:

- the ear lobe
- the bodies of the cervical vertebrae (the neck)
- the tip of the shoulder
- dividing the thorax (ribcage) in half
- the bodies of the lumbar vertebrae
- slightly behind the hip joint
- slightly in front of the centre of the knee joint
- slightly in front of the outside ankle bone (lateral malleolus)

This diagram below illustrates what we mean by good posture.

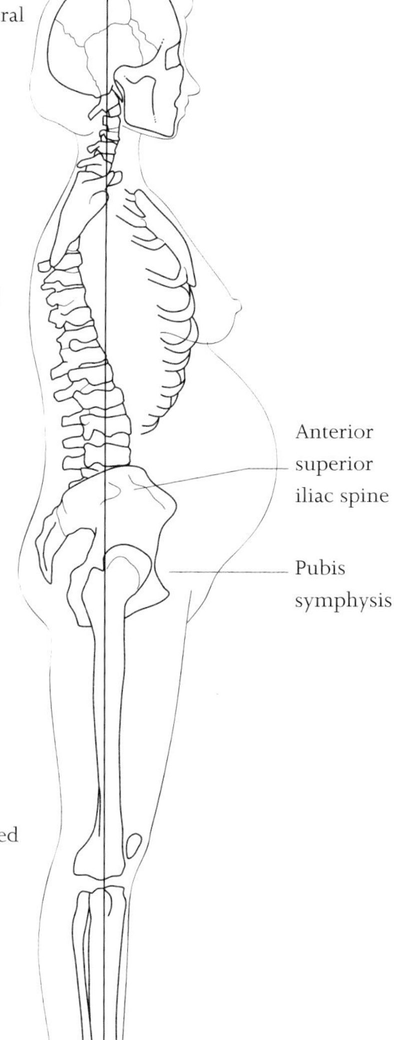

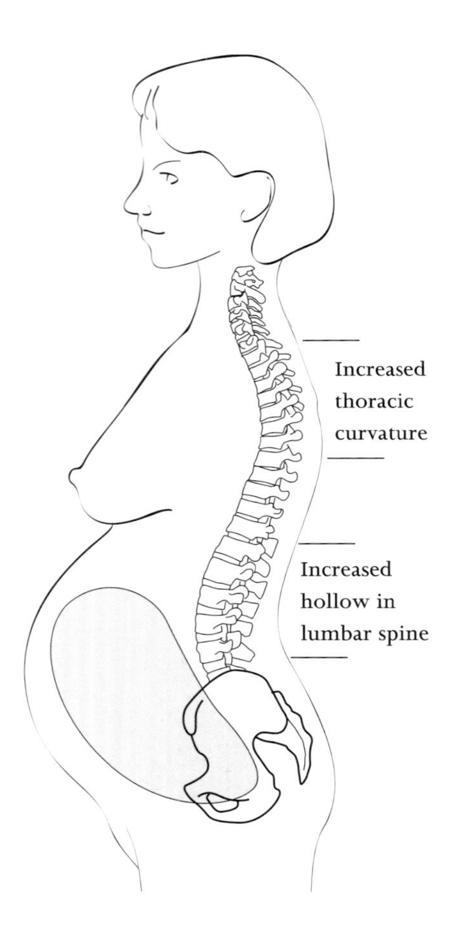

On average, a pregnant woman will put on about 13.8 kilos (30 pounds) by the time she reaches full term. This is not all baby, thank heavens! It is the combined weight of the baby, the placenta, the uterus, the amniotic fluid, increased breast tissue, increased blood volume, fat stores and increased tissue fluids. It is the increased weight of the breasts and uterus, combined with the weight of the baby and the extra fluid that has the greatest effect on your posture. Your centre of gravity is going to shift and no longer fall over the feet. Usually you correct this automatically by leaning back. Looking at the typical pregnancy stance, you can see the increased curvature in the upper back (kyphosis) caused by the weight of the breasts, the resulting increased curve in the neck and the increased hollow in the lumbar spine (lordosis) due to the increased weight of the uterus and the resulting forward tilt of the pelvis, but not all women adopt this stance.

Stand side on to a mirror or ask a friend to check your posture. Does it match this diagram? Most likely it will, but not always. Do not assume that your body will adjust to the shift in gravity in this way. **Each woman is different.** With some mothers the pelvis tilts posteriorly and the lumbar curve flattens. In this case, you will have to take extra care to maintain a curve in the lumbar spine while exercising, standing and sitting.

If you wish to avoid the aches and pains associated with muscle tension and joint misalignment, it is even more important during your pregnancy that you learn how to stand and sit well. This is not just for when you are doing your Pilates session but for all your daily activities.

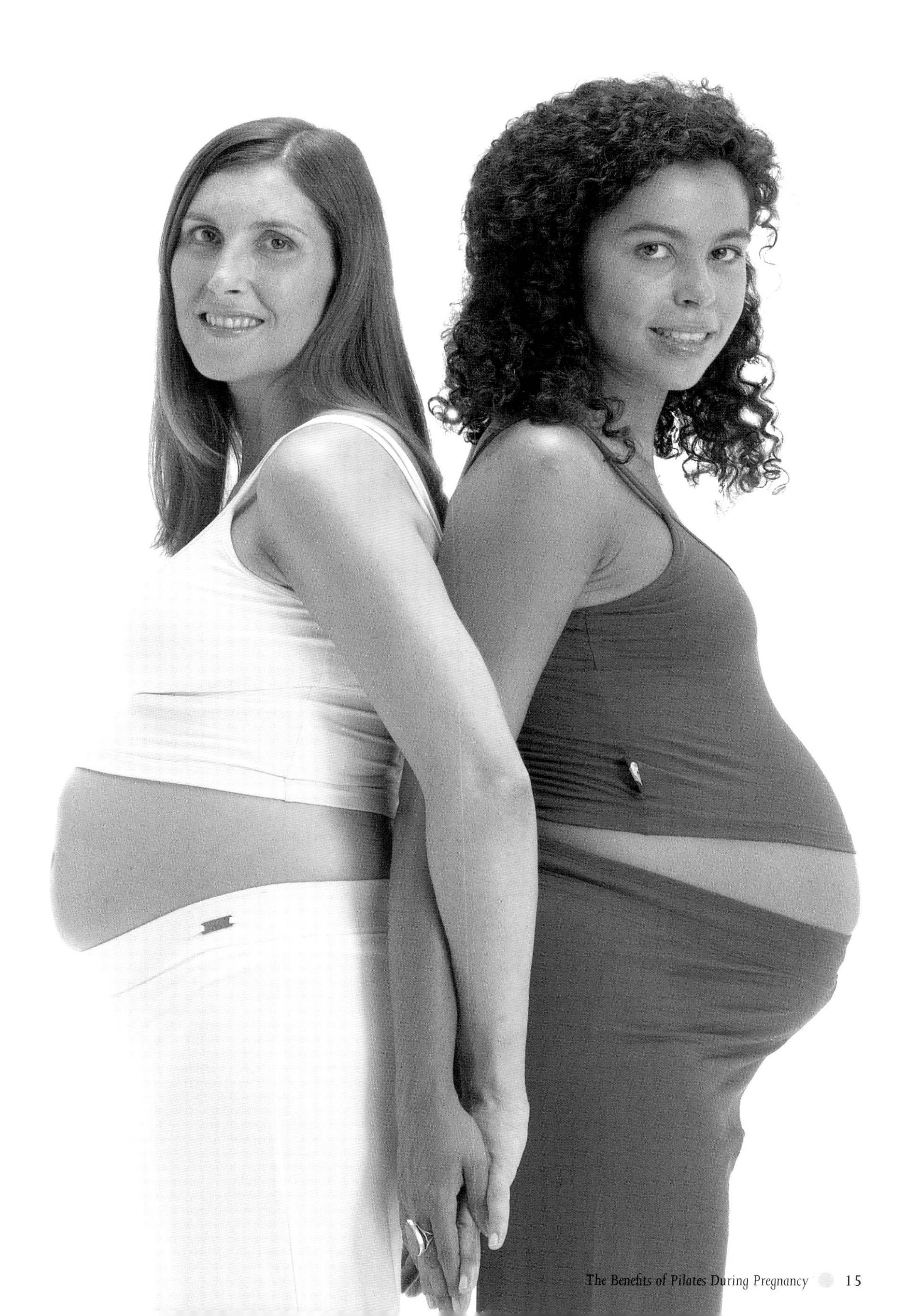

Standing Well

- Stand comfortably with your feet hip-width apart. They should either be in parallel or with a natural slight turn-out if this is comfortable.
- Imagine a balloon attached to the top of your head lifting you up through the spine.
- Allow your neck to release.
- Allow your shoulder blades to widen and your collarbones to open in front of the chest.
- Allow your ribcage to relax.
- Have your palms facing the seams of your trousers.
- Soften your armpits, and direct your elbows away.
- Lengthen up out of your hips, but do not force this.
- Check that the pelvis is in neutral (page 46) and that the muscles at the front of the hips are soft. Imagine a weight attached to your tailbone (coccyx) allowing it to drop down, anchoring but not tilting it.
- Release your knees.
- Are your feet hip-width apart? Keep the weight evenly balanced on both feet – do not allow them to roll in or out. Your feet should be firmly anchored to the floor through the base of the big toes, the base of the small toes and the centre of the heels.
- Now focus on allowing the head to balance freely over the ribcage, which is floating over the hips. The hips float over the feet.
- You are at once grounded through the soles of your feet, yet lengthening up through your spine.
- Keep the three main body weights, head, ribcage and pelvis balanced over each other and centrally over the legs.

Please avoid the regular wearing of high heels while you are pregnant. They tend to throw the pelvis forward. Save them for special occasions.

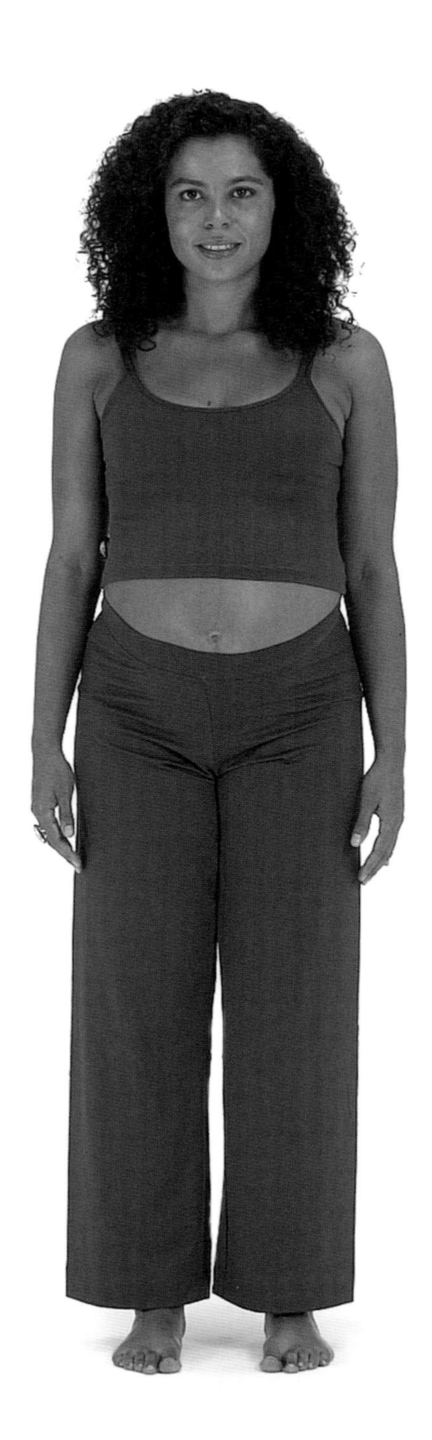

Good Posture When Sitting

The single most important thing to remember when seated is to keep the natural 'S' curve of the spine (see page 13). Do not allow yourself to sink back into a 'C' curve.

Chairs or sofas that are too soft, too low or too deep will not encourage you to sit well. Initially they might feel relaxing, but this is short-lived.

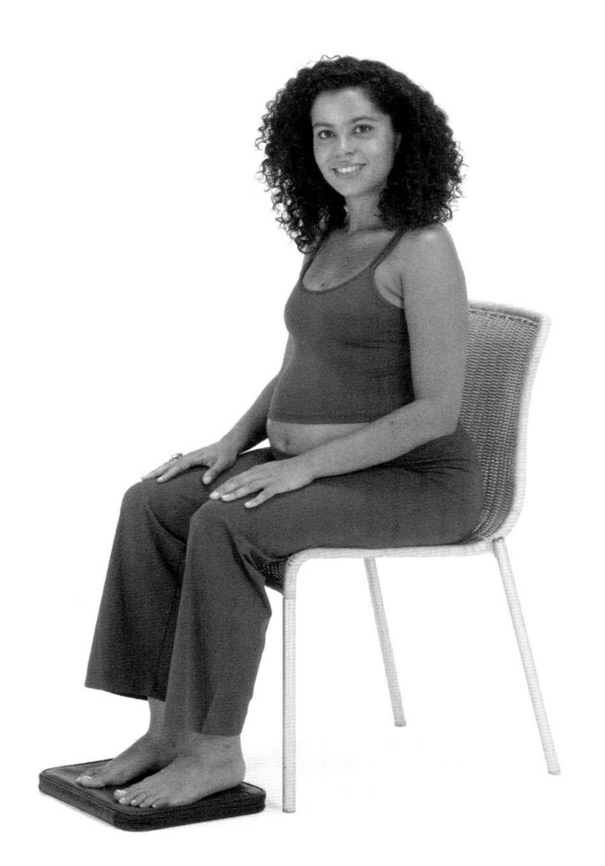

Sitting Well

- Sit on your sitting bones. You can feel these when you sit on a hard chair and place your hands under each buttock. By transferring your weight from cheek to cheek, you can feel the sitting bones. The weight should be evenly distributed between those bones. Try to keep your pelvis in neutral (page 46–7).
- Your feet should be planted firmly on the floor, hip-width apart.
- When sitting on normal chairs where the seat is parallel to the floor try to keep the lower part of your legs at 90° to the thighs. The height of the chair is, therefore, very important. If it is too high your feet will be dangling. In this case, a footstool or a telephone directory can help to alleviate this problem. If the seat is too low – as with some sofas – you are increasing the pressure on the lower back because it is much harder to maintain the natural curves of the spine.
- The back of your knee should be 5 centimetres (2 inches) away from the seat edge so as not to restrict blood circulation to the lower leg.
- Avoid crossing your legs because this twists your spine and restricts circulation in the legs.
- Keep your back long with its natural 'S' curve still present. When you are slouching you are making a 'C' curve and are, therefore, increasing the pressure on joints and discs.
- If you are working at a desk, do not perch too far forward on the edge of the chair.
- Supporting the lower (lumbar) back is sometimes necessary, especially if your core stabilizing muscles are not yet strong enough to do the job. A good chair provides this support, but a lumbar roll or a small cushion can be equally as effective – and you can take them wherever you are going!
- Relax your shoulders and thighs.
- Avoid sitting for long periods of time. Move about every half an hour to stretch the back and decrease the pressure.
- The position of your head is very important. It is very heavy and can pull the spine out of alignment. Keep your neck soft and tension free.

Choosing a Chair for Sitting at Work

There are now many companies that specialize in ergonomically designed office chairs (see Further Information, page 184). Here are the most important things to look out for:

- Choose a chair where you can adjust the seat height and angle.
- Ideally your thighs should be sloping downwards. For this the chair seat needs to have a forward slope of 5–15° so that your hips are slightly higher than your knees. This is perfect, but not always possible. If you work at a desk then it is worth investing in a really good chair (or asking your employer to).
- Altering the angle of the seat during the day is very beneficial. A 5° angle is ideal. Posture wedges can also alter the angle of the seat.
- Back support is crucial and should also be adjustable to allow lumbar support.
- Armrests need to be exactly the right height, otherwise they can prevent you from sitting well. They should be able to go under the desk, otherwise you are too far away from the workstation. They should support your arms, but not encourage you to lift your shoulders.
- Swivel chairs are beneficial because you can change position without twisting your back.

Your Workstation

The height of the desk is as important as the height of the chair. To determine the right height, bear in mind that, when working on a personal computer, your forearms and wrists should be parallel with or slightly sloping downwards to the desk.

The height of the computer screen is also crucial. The top line of text on the screen should be level with your eyes. You should not have to look down to see the screen because this causes tension in the neck and back. Propping the screen up with books can be useful. The legs should be under the desk so you do not have to reach forward to the keyboard. The desk should therefore be quite deep.

Avoid cradling the telephone in your neck! Keep both shoulder blades down and your neck released. If you are a heavy telephone user, use a headset or, if circumstances allow, a hands-free telephone.

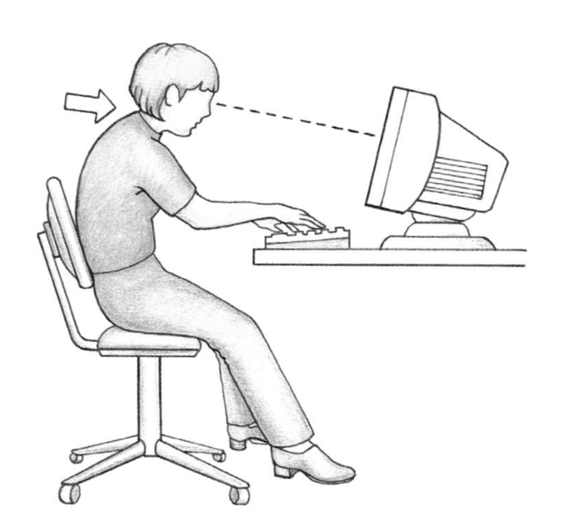

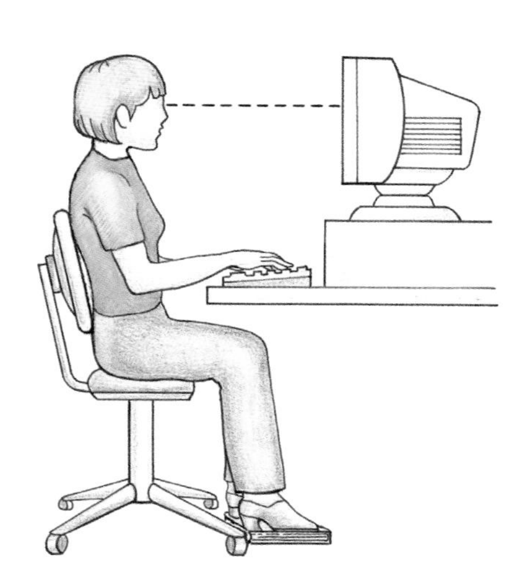

Getting Up from a Chair

When you get up from a chair, place your feet hip-width apart, but with one foot slightly in front of the other. Lean forward over your legs and, keeping the natural curves in your back and not allowing it to overarch or hollow, lengthen through the top of the head and rise up using your thigh and back muscles.

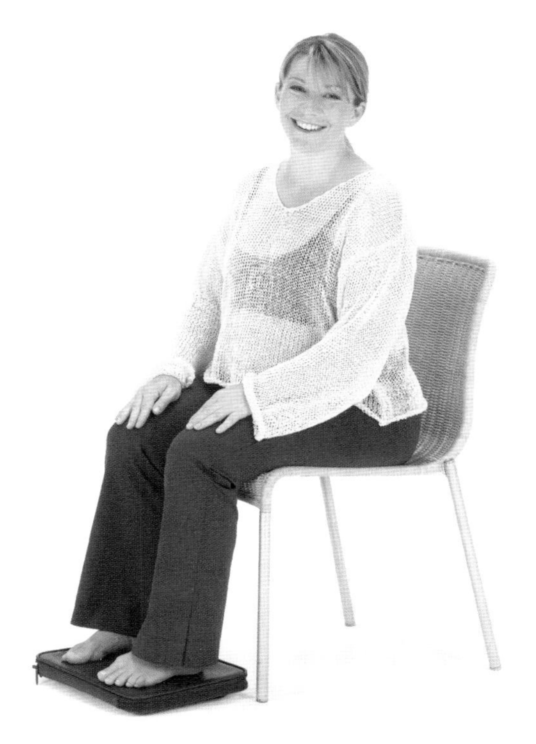

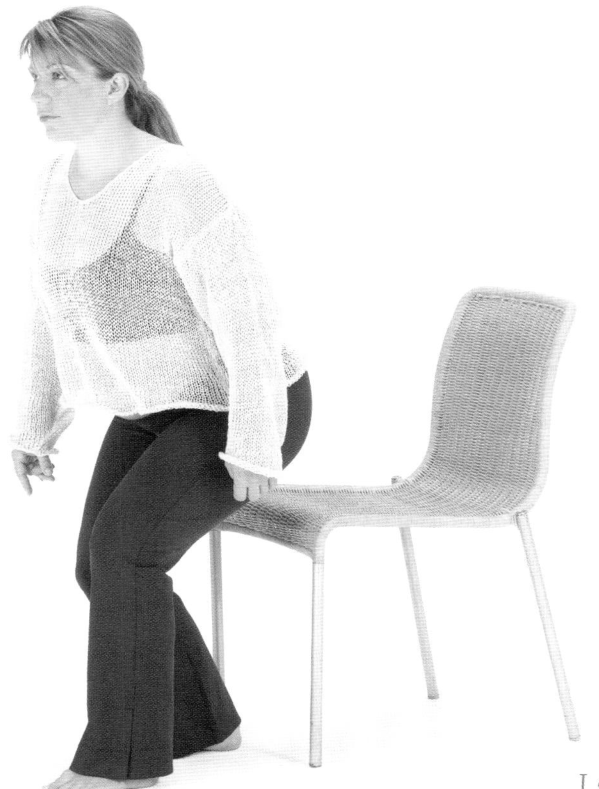

I started doing Pilates about nine years ago, and have carried on doing it, except when a period of serious illness prevented me. Pilates helped my recovery and I am now expecting a baby in May, something I was told would be impossible for me. I have already ordered the new Pilates for Pregnancy video and am really looking forward to it. – H. Cunniffe

Sleeping Well

A good night's rest is vital to a healthy pregnant or non-pregnant body. It is while you sleep that a lot of the body's repair work at cellular level takes place, and the body therefore regenerates itself.

The choice of bed is important. It should support you properly. If the mattress is too soft, your back will not be supported, and if it is too hard and does not give at the shoulders and hips, you will lose the natural curves of your spine. The bigger the bed the more space you have to move around so you are less likely to sleep in one awkward position. If you naturally tend to sleep on your back, you will probably find that as your uterus grows this position will become increasingly uncomfortable and may even make you feel dizzy and nauseous (see page 118).

Prolonged sleeping on your stomach (not an option later in the pregnancy) can strain your back and a cushion under your abdomen can alleviate this or you could or you could try using a 'belly bag'. A wonderful new piece of furniture designed for pregnancy which allows you to lie on your front. (See Further Information on page 184 for stockists.)

Sleeping on your side is usually the best option. Make sure you keep your spine aligned (see below). A pillow between your knees can make you more comfortable (and another under your bump). Sleeping on your left side is particularly beneficial.

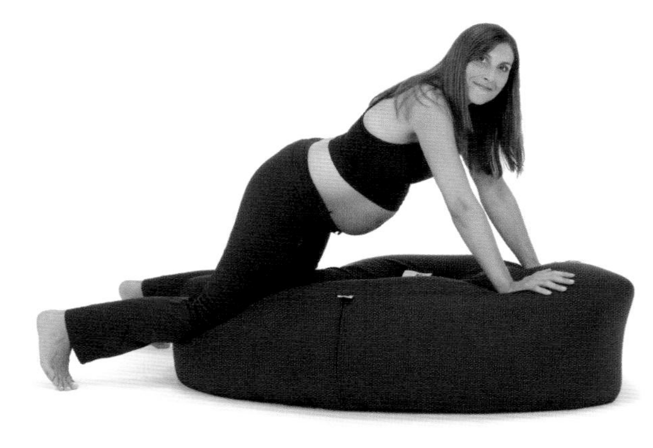

The belly bag

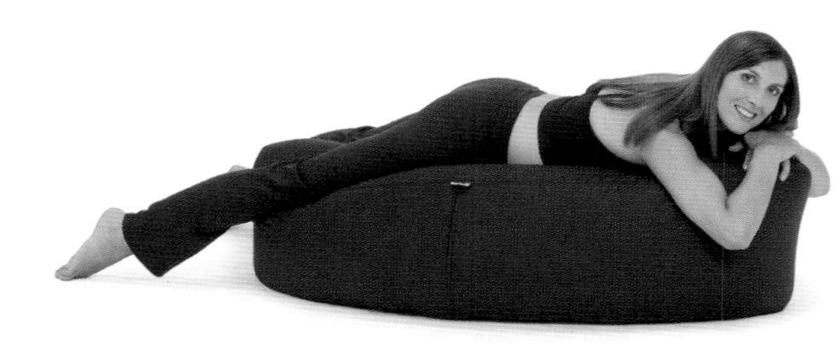

✓

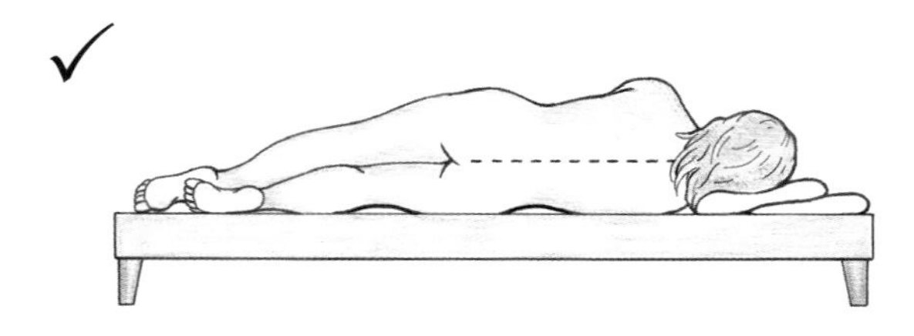

✗

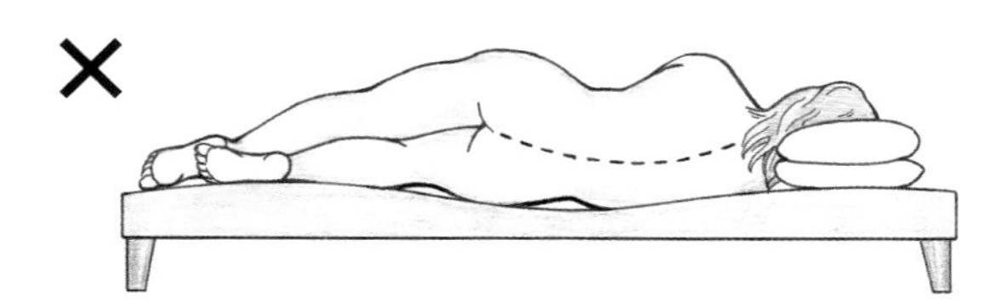

Lifting and Carrying Well

It is inevitable that during your pregnancy you will still have to lift and carry either young children or heavy shopping. You should avoid lifting very heavy objects while pregnant, but if you have to lift something heavy follow the advice given opposite and do not twist! Please bear in mind that you will not have these guidelines with you at the time, so you need to practise the movements now.

- Where possible, take the time to divide the load. It may take a little longer to complete the task, but it is better than harming your back. Do not be afraid to ask someone to help you. An extra pair of hands will lighten the weight.
- When you are about to lift something, it is important to position yourself correctly to start with.
- You should be aware of the weight of the object you are about to lift.
- Stand as close as possible to the load and have your feet on either side of it, with one foot slightly in front of the other, just as if you were taking a step.
- Bend at the knees and hips to squat down. This is something like doing Monkey Bends on page 129.
- Keep your back long and strongly supported by zipping up and hollowing (pages 48–56).
- Keeping your body close to the load, use the handles or place one hand under the object and the other hand on top.
- As you lift, make sure you keep the load close to your body. The further away you hold it, the more you are straining your back.
- Lean forward and, while maintaining a long back, straighten your knees and hips.
- Avoid lifting and twisting at the same time. Lift first and then rotate the whole trunk round to where you want to go.

When Is It Not Safe to Exercise?

IMPORTANT NOTE

If you are having twins (or more!), you must seek medical advice as to whether you may follow this programme.

The following guidelines relate to cardiovascular exercise, but if you suffer from any of the following, you may be advised by your doctor not to do Pilates exercise:

severe anaemia

cardiac arrhythmia

chronic bronchitis

type 1 diabetes

extreme obesity

extreme underweight

intrauterine growth restriction in current pregnancy

orthopaedic limitations

poorly controlled seizure disorder

poorly controlled thyroid disease

or if you are a heavy smoker

Contraindications to Exercise in Pregnancy

- three or more miscarriages
- maternal heart disease
- maternal diabetes
- pain
- bleeding
- high blood pressure
- fever
- if you suffer from severe headaches, especially if they are accompanied by swelling, blurring of vision or pain at the side of the ribcage, see your GP immediately, because these symptoms could indicate pre-eclampsia (toxaemia), a condition characterized by high blood pressure, swelling and protein in the urine which, if untreated, can lead to eclampsia, a serious but very rare condition which can prove fatal for mother and baby
- incompetent cervix where the neck of the womb opens prematurely due to the pressure on it of the uterus and the baby
- placenta praevia where the placenta is attached to the lower half of the uterus, covering or partially covering the opening of the cervix – because exercise may exacerbate bleeding.

The Risk of Miscarriage

One in four women will have a miscarriage; the first three months and in particular the first 8–14 weeks is when most miscarriages occur, so this is a time for caution. If you have been practising Pilates before you became pregnant and if your practitioner agrees (please see the list of contraindications to exercise), you may continue with a gentle Pilates programme during this time, but you will need to adapt your workouts, following the guidelines given on pages 98 and 121 (note that this period goes from the end of the first trimester to the beginning of the second trimester). Ultimately, the decision whether to continue exercising or not rests with you and your doctor. We can only offer general advice. If you are at all apprehensive, then wait until after 16 weeks, when the pregnancy is well established.

If you are new to Pilates we recommend you wait until after 16 weeks before you start the programme.

If you have not done Pilates before, you will need to learn the basic exercises in Chapter 5. Once you have mastered these, you can start with the exercises given in Chapter 8 on the second trimester, bearing in mind that you will need to learn any recommended exercises from the earlier chapters, Preparing for Your Pregnancy and The First Trimester.

When to Stop Exercising

If at any time during your pregnancy you experience any of the following, do not continue with the exercises and immediately seek medical advice. If:

- your membranes have ruptured
- you are in pain
- you are bleeding
- you are very short of breath
- you feel dizzy, faint and/or disorientated
- you develop tachycardia – a fast or an irregular heart beat
- you have pubic pain
- you have difficulty in walking
- your blood pressure is high
- you develop severe headaches accompanied by swelling, blurring of vision, pain at the side of the ribcage; see your GP immediately because these symptoms could indicate pre-eclampsia (page 22)
- you are unwell or have a fever
- you are very anaemic
- you develop phlebitis or blood clots
- you have a breech in your third trimester, seek advice; sometimes exercise is used to turn the baby, but you will need medical guidance as to which exercises are suitable
- you haven't felt the baby move – you should feel at least ten movements per twelve waking hours. In the second trimester after the quickening, the baby's movements will be quite vigorous but as the baby grows in the third trimester and has less space to move, the movements will feel more like he or she is squirming
- your pulse stays elevated after exercise (this is more relevant for cardiovascular work)
- you develop swelling, pain or tenderness in the calf or leg

2 What Is Pilates?

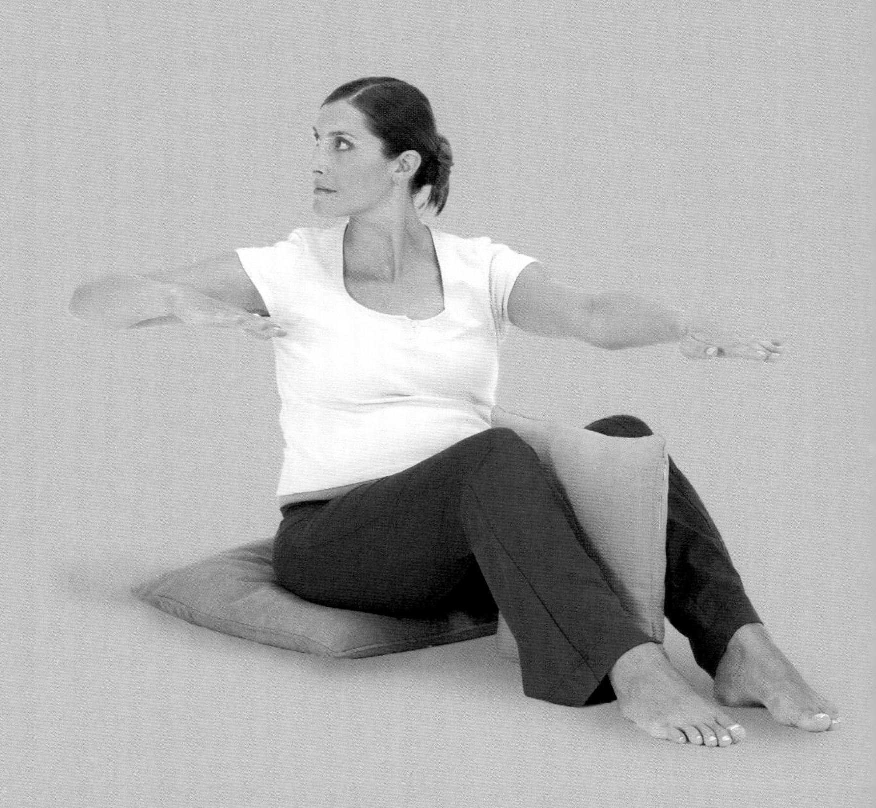

The Eight Principles of Body Control Pilates

There are Eight Principles behind the Body Control Pilates Method:

- relaxation
- concentration
- alignment
- breathing
- centring
- co-ordination
- flowing movements
- stamina

Relaxation

There is a wonderful line in *The Bonesetter's Daughter* by Amy Tan when the main character Ruth talks about her favourite form of exercise, 'Stress – you clench your muscles for twelve hours, release for a count of five, then clench again.' Sound familiar? Most of us suffer from some form of stress. Pregnancy is a time when you have a lot to cope with, and because of your hormonal imbalance you can feel emotionally very unstable. Next time you feel yourself under pressure, stop and take note of which parts of the body are tense – jaw? neck? shoulders? back? Those tight knots the masseur's fingers so expertly probe – that sweet agony as the kinks unwind. It is often very hard for these muscles to release, and not stay switched on. Therefore, one of our first priorities is to help you learn how to switch them off and make sure that everyday stress isn't brought into an exercise session. But by relaxed we do not mean collapsed. We need you ready to exercise and to move freely using the right muscles to make the movements. Being able to release unnecessary tension will also prove invaluable during labour.

The Relaxation Position is a good way to start a session and we use it as the starting and finishing position for many of the exercises as well.

IMPORTANT NOTE

You should not remain in this position for longer than 3 minutes in your second and third trimesters.

The Relaxation Position

Lie flat on your back with a small towel or firm, flat pillow underneath your head, if necessary, to allow the back of the neck to lengthen. Keep your feet parallel and hip-width apart, that is in a line with the centre of your buttocks. Have your knees bent. Place your hands on your lower abdomen. In this position you can easily run through a checklist. Ask yourself:

- Am I holding tension in my neck and shoulders? If so, allow your neck to soften and your shoulders to widen and melt into the mat.
- Does my low back feel tight? Check that you have kept the natural curves of your spine (see opposite), then allow the spine to lengthen. Imagine you have dry sand in your back pockets and allow it to gently trickle out.
- Is my pelvis in neutral? Is my sacrum square on the mat? If necessary, go through the Compass (page 46).
- Are my thighs tense? You may have to adjust where you place your feet, bringing them nearer to your bottom or taking them further away.
- Have I got my knees in a line with my hips? Try lining them up with the middle of each buttock cheek.
- Can I feel the three points on the soles of my feet in contact with the floor – base of the big toes, base of the small toes, centre of the heels?

When you have completed your checklist, you can start the exercise session confident that your alignment is good and you have let go of any unnecessary tension. However, you will need to remain vigilant while you perform the exercises or those overactive, dominant muscles will kick back in.

Concentration

Hand in hand with relaxation goes concentration. It is a sad fact that due to hormonal changes while you are pregnant your ability to focus and concentrate may diminish. You can become rather scatterbrained. Pilates is a mental and physical conditioning programme that should help train both your mind and your body. Because it requires you to focus on each movement made, it develops your body's sensory feedback, or proprioception, so that you know where you are in space and what you are doing with every part of your body for every second you are moving. Although the movements themselves may become automatic with time, you still have to concentrate, because there is always a further level of awareness to reach.

Use the exercises in this book to train your mind–body connection and you will find that you are far more body aware not just when you exercise but in your daily activities. You will be able to concentrate better and will be far more co-ordinated in your movements. Learn to listen to the natural intelligence of your body – it really does talk to you!

IMPORTANT NOTE

You should not remain in this position for longer than 3 minutes in your second and third trimesters.

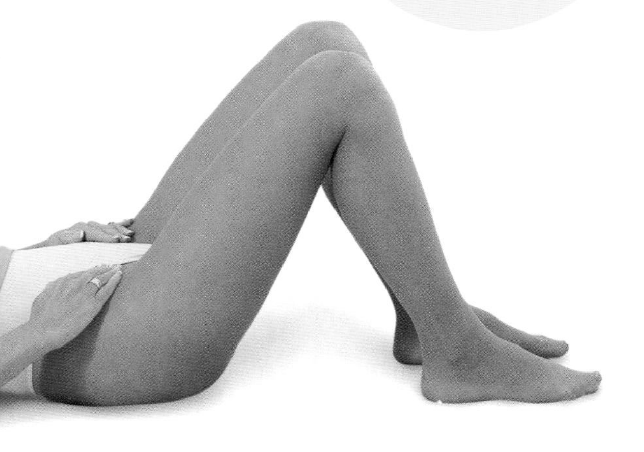

Alignment

We have already seen how your posture is going to change during pregnancy. By constantly reminding your body of how it should be standing, sitting or lying and by moving correctly, you can bring it into good postural alignment. This is essential not only to restore muscle balance and prevent aches and pains but also so you look good. If you exercise without concern for the correct position of the joints, you risk stressing them, which can lead to extra wear and tear. Muscles have an optimal length at which they function best – if you have poor postural alignment this length may have been altered and the muscles may be too long or too short. Either way, their ability to do their job properly is affected. By placing your bones in the right place before you start an exercise and being aware of where they are while you do the exercise, you stand a good chance of getting the right muscles working (good movement), which means your workout is going to be really effective.

What we are aiming for is that you are able to recognize and keep your joints in their 'neutral' positions – that is in the ideal position for good muscle balance and healthy ligaments. Gradually, your body will 'remember' the positions – you will find yourself sitting correctly and walking taller.

Refer back to the checklists for the Relaxation Position on the opposite page and for Standing Well (page 16) and Sitting Well (page 17).

Many of our exercises require you to have your spine and pelvis in their natural neutral positions. For the spine, this means the position where it keeps its length and its natural 'S' shape. This is the position where there is least stress on the facet joints (at the back of the vertebrae), the ligaments and the discs, and which allows the muscles to be at their optimal length and so function normally when we move.

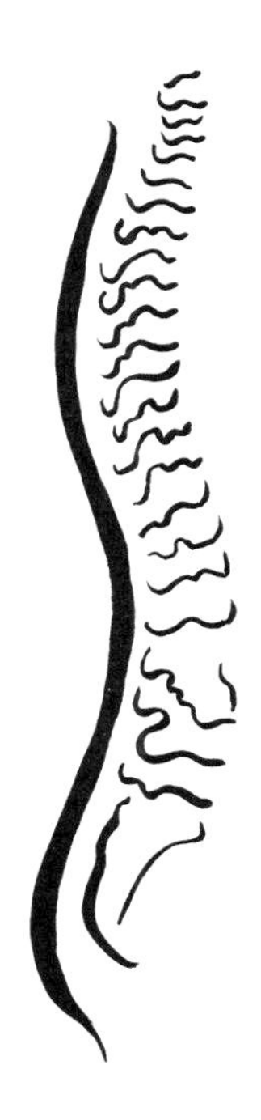

The Compass on page 46 is designed to help you find the correct neutral position of the pelvis and the spine.

Please remember that good alignment refers to the whole body; how you place your hands, your feet, your head, neck and shoulders while doing the exercises will all contribute to good posture. Pay close attention to the directions given in each exercise. A misplaced foot may prevent your pelvis from being in neutral. A tilted head can cause muscle tension. Good hand, wrist, elbow and shoulder alignment can help prevent carpal tunnel syndrome (see page 118).

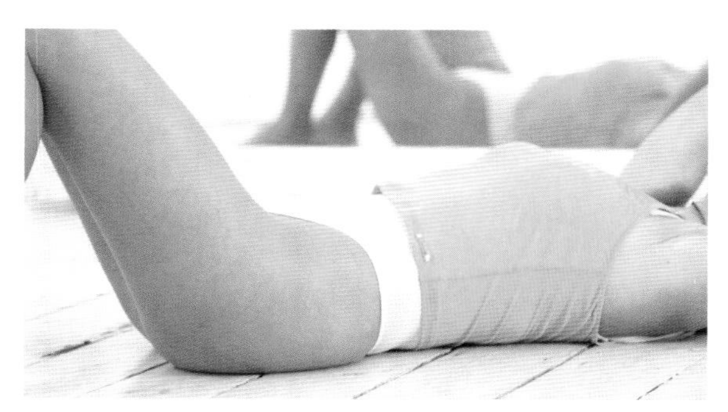

Neutral

Breathing

Improving your breathing is probably the single most dramatic difference you can make to your overall health – yet it is the one thing that we all take for granted. Few of us breathe efficiently, and what a waste that is because we miss out on all that wonderful oxygen which nourishes and replenishes every cell in the body and also has an important role to play in burning calories and shedding fat. We may go to great expense to buy the latest oxygen-rich skin creams or even spend time in oxygen tents, but the best results are to be had by simply learning to breathe more effectively, increasing the lung capacity, and using the lower as well as the upper lobes of the lungs. By taking the time to master lateral or thoracic breathing, you can ultimately improve your overall well-being. What's more, once this breathing becomes automatic, once it becomes your natural subconscious way of breathing, you reap the benefits every second of the day and night.

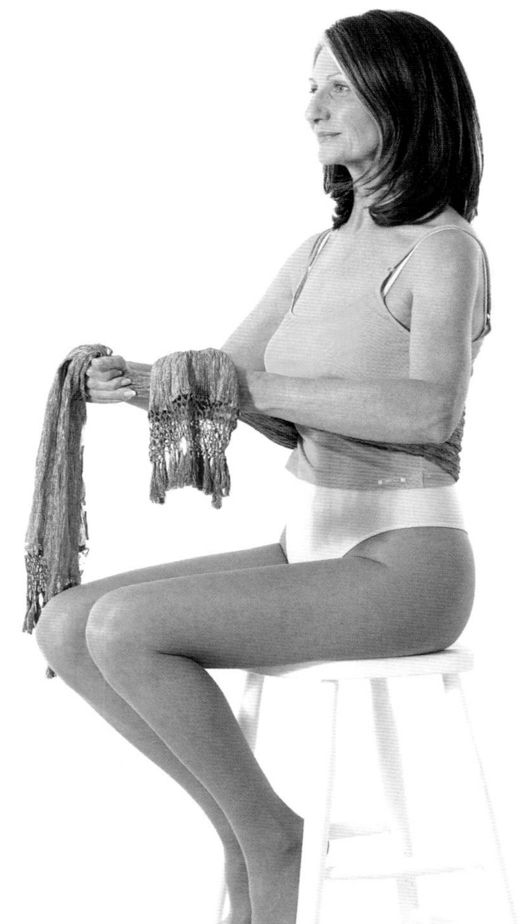

Centring: Creating a Girdle of Strength

Joseph Pilates had no formal medical training but he discovered that if he hollowed his navel back towards his spine, the low back felt protected and he thus introduced the direction 'navel to spine' for all his exercises. He called the area between the hips and the ribcage 'the powerhouse' and taught that all movements should originate from this strong centre – this natural girdle of strength. In so doing he was using the deep postural muscles to stabilize the spine – physiotherapists today call this 'core stability'. The key muscles are transversus abdominis the deepest of your abdominal muscles and multifidus, a deep spinal muscle.

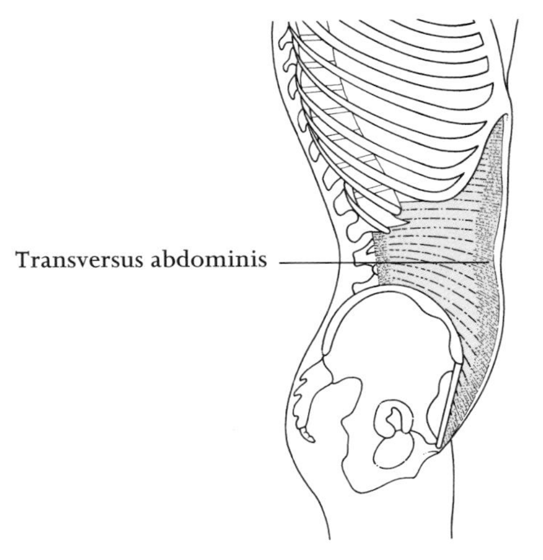

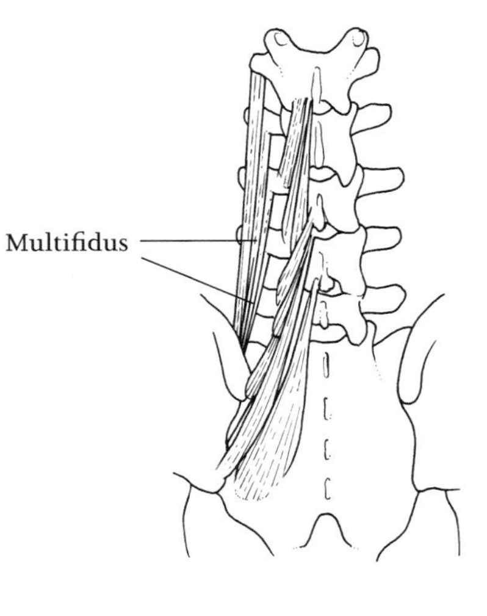

Think of the vertebrae of your spine being like a pile of books, stacked one on top of the other. The role of transversus and multifidus is to prevent one of the books slipping out of place, in other words, to prevent one vertebra slipping too far off its neighbour, which can cause everything from facet joint to disc problems. Unfortunately, poor posture, sitting for long periods of time and slouching, often mean that the deep stabilizing muscles are held lengthened and under stress. Add to this the extra weight of your growing uterus, the trauma of labour, carrying a baby badly (usually on one hip!), lack of exercise, or the wrong type of exercise, and it is easy to see why these deep postural muscles are weakened.

The exercises on pages 48 to 56 will teach you how to locate and strengthen your deep stabilizing muscles with the zip up and hollow action.

Once you have learnt to create a strong centre, we can start to challenge that stability by moving the limbs and adding movements such rotation, flexion and lateral flexion and extension. A good workout should include all these movements.

What we are aiming for is free-flowing movements around a strong base. Bear in mind that all joints in the body have stabilizing muscles whose role it is to fix and hold the bones in place, allowing the more superficial (mobilizing) muscles to execute the movements. When these deep stabilizing muscles are weak, the balance of the muscles is upset, and the more superficial movement muscles have to take on the stabilizing role.

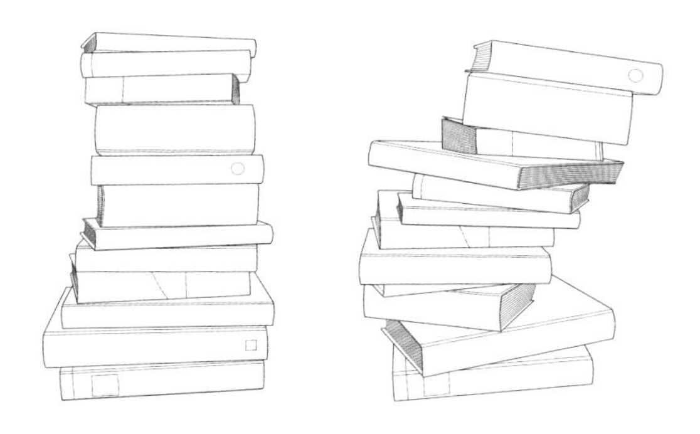

Transversus and multifidus keep the vertebra stacked and stable like a neat pile of books

For example, if you find your hamstrings are really tight despite a lot of stretching it may be that they are shortened because they are having to stabilize the pelvis because the muscles which should be stabilizing the pelvis are weak (that is transversus and the deep gluteals). Similarly, if your low back feels tight it may be that the erector spinae muscle group (primarily mobilizing muscles) are having to do the work that the deep stabilizing muscles (transversus abdominals and multifidus) are not doing properly.

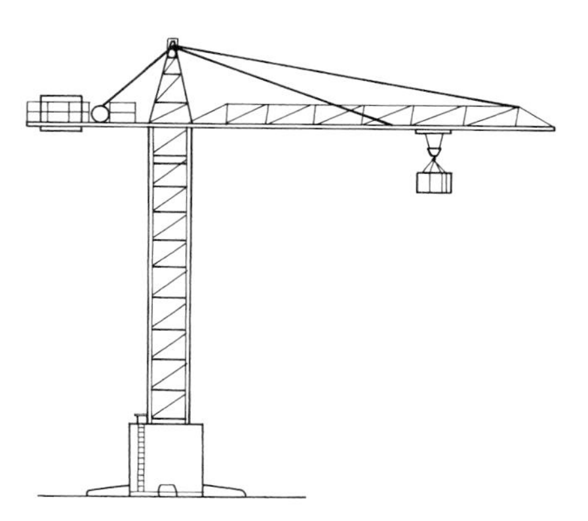

Imagine a tower crane on a building site. The base of the crane represents the deep postural stabilizing muscles holding and supporting the arm of the crane (the mobilizing muscles). For the crane to be stable while the arm lifts heavy weights and makes large swinging movements, the base must be strong. If the balance is upset, the crane will not function properly and may topple.

It is exactly the same with your body and, remember, there is even more strain on the skeletal frame and muscles when you are pregnant. If your deep stabilizing muscles aren't supporting your joints because they are too weak, your movement patterns are upset and your joints are placed under strain. This is why we aim to build strength from the inside out. First we must learn how to position the body correctly then we need to strengthen the deep postural muscles. Once we have done this, we can learn good movement skills and then go on to strengthen the rest of the body.

Co-ordination

So, now you are relaxed, focused, aware and aligned, you are breathing efficiently (or learning to) and you have located and strengthened your deep core muscles, you are therefore ready to add movement. Step by step the exercises will teach you how to move well. It may seem strange to begin with; it will feel different (after all you have probably been moving badly for many years), but the movements soon become automatic, ingrained or 'grooved' as they are locked into the body's memory. Meanwhile, the actual process of learning these new co-ordination skills is excellent mental and physical training, stimulating the two-way communication channel between mind and body.

When you are pregnant the male hormone testosterone decreases. Testosterone affects your hand to eye co-ordination and your sense of balance. Pilates is a wonderful way of countering this, helping you feel more balanced, co-ordinated and confident in your movements.

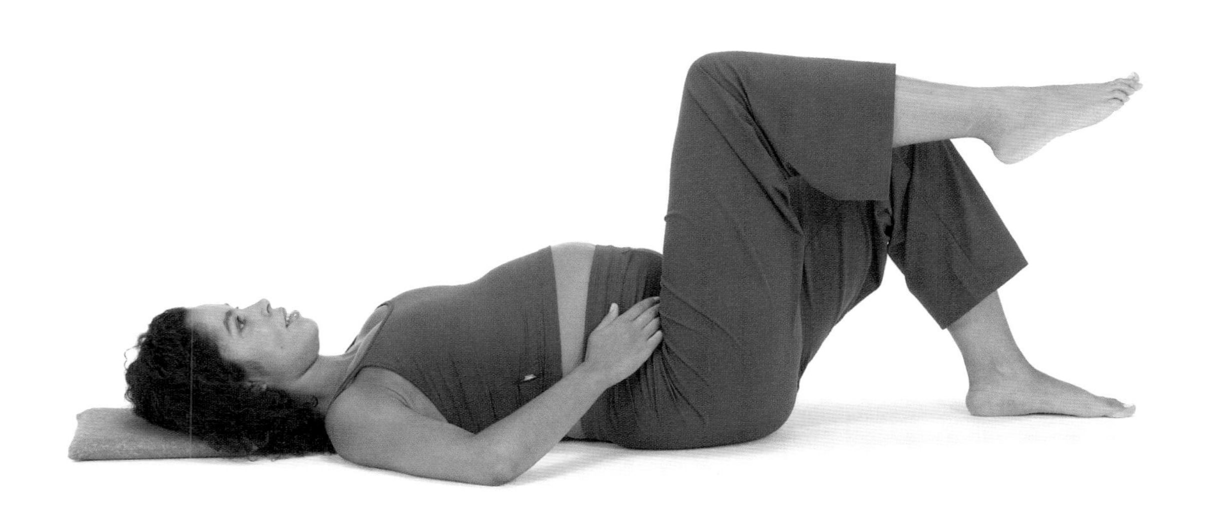

Flowing Movements

Pilates is about natural movements performed smoothly, gracefully and with attention to detail. You will not be required to twist into awkward positions or to strain. We start with small movements and build up to more complicated combinations – the idea is to be constantly challenged. When you are a beginner you need to keep your limbs close to you, rather than risk losing your alignment and stability, but as you grow more confident and proficient you take your joints through their full range of motion. When you are pregnant, due to your joint instability, we will limit your ranges of motion somewhat, but the movements will still be natural and free flowing. Whatever exercise you are performing, the movements must be precisely executed with control. The movements are generally slow, lengthening away from a strong centre, which gives you the opportunity to check your alignment and focus on using the right muscles. Slow doesn't mean easy though – in fact it is harder to do an exercise slowly than quickly and it is also less easy to cheat!

Stamina

Stamina is going to be one of your greatest requirements as your pregnancy progresses and during labour itself. Many pregnant women complain of tiredness after a day on their feet, simply because standing badly is tiring: the ribcage is compressed and as a consequence, the lungs are constricted. As you learn to open and lengthen the body, breathing becomes more efficient. All Pilates exercises are designed to encourage the respiratory, lymphatic and circulatory systems to function more effectively. As you become more proficient at the exercises and your muscles begin to strengthen and work correctly, you will discover that your overall stamina improves dramatically. You will no longer be wasting energy holding on to unnecessary tension or moving inefficiently. Your body will move as nature intended. You will be fit for labour and beyond!

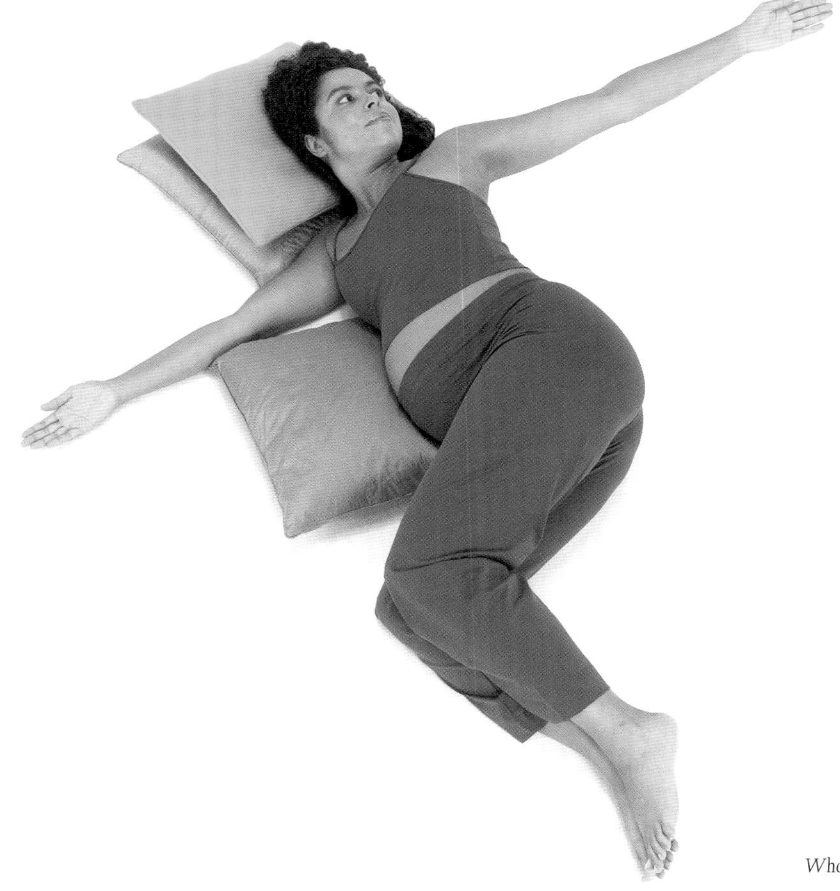

Joseph Pilates and the Origins of the Pilates Method

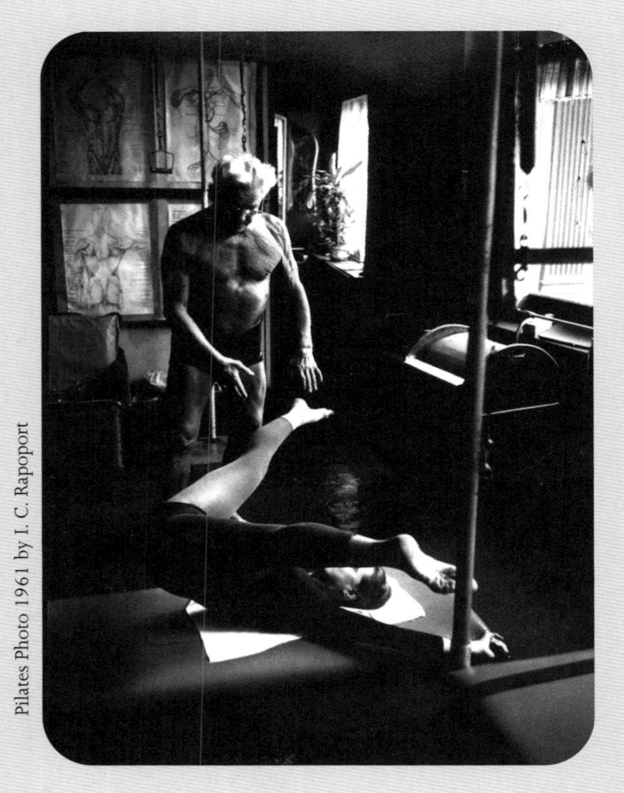

Pilates Photo 1961 by I. C. Rapoport

The Pilates Method was developed by the late Joseph Hubertus Pilates. Born in Germany in 1880, he overcame a childhood that was plagued by ill health and, perhaps as a consequence, became obsessed with physical fitness to improve his body image. He was a keen sportsman, and many elements from his range of interests, including martial arts and gymnastics, found their way into a fitness programme that he initially devised for his fellow internees while he was interned in England during the First World War.

He returned to Germany after the war and made a living teaching self-defence and fitness to the police and the army. He moved, in 1926, to the USA to distance himself from unfolding events in Germany and proceeded to set up a fitness studio in New York, at an address he shared with the New York City Ballet. His first clients were boxers, but he was soon working with leading ballet dancers, actors, actresses and athletes because his exercises were felt to perfect and complement their traditional exercise programmes. He struck a strange figure, often teaching in his swimming trunks and not afraid to give very robust correction to clients during exercises. But his ideas and approach have been shown to be years ahead of their time because, today, the Pilates Method is a core part of the training programme for a wide range of elite athletes and performers, and is also supported by medical specialists.

Joseph Pilates died in 1967, his death being caused indirectly by the effects of a fire at his studio. His legacy was to leave a method of body conditioning that was never precisely laid down, but which has been developed and expanded by teachers since then.

The Development of Body Control Pilates

The Body Control Pilates Method is closely based on the work of Joseph Pilates, and is unique in the way that it prepares the body for what are known as the 'classical' Pilates exercises, many of which are far too advanced for the average person new to Pilates.

Our approach is based on the belief that the necessary skills and movements should be taught progressively, building layer upon layer towards the end result of performing the intermediate and advanced exercises safely and effectively. We have also broken the exercises down so they can be done by an 'average body', rather than just by people who come from the worlds of dance or sport, the traditional sources of Pilates enthusiasts. It is this approach that has won the support of many of the leading medical bodies and of several athletes and governing bodies in sport.

The Body Control Pilates programme was developed in 1996 by Lynne Robinson and Gordon Thomson and, ahead of the publication of Lynne and Gordon's first book *Body Control the Pilates Way* in March 1997 (a book of which there were only humble expectations, yet which quickly became an international exercise bestseller), we established our first training course for those wanting to learn to teach the Body Control Pilates Method.

Seven years on, it is hard to remember just what pioneering days those were. Today, Pilates is one of the most popular exercise regimes. Barely a week goes by without a 'celebrity mention' in the national media, and Body Control Pilates is the in-flight exercise programme for British Airways, is promotionally linked with major consumer brands such as Kelloggs, and is used by the Great British rowing team. You will probably also find a qualified teacher close to you, because the Body Control Pilates Association now has more than 600 members, all of whom have undergone extensive training to gain certification to teach the Body Control Pilates Method. To retain this certification, Body Control Pilates teachers also have to undertake further professional development studies every year.

Lynne Robinson and Jacqueline Knox (medical consultant for this book) have together developed a very popular Pilates for Pregnancy course for Pilates teachers.

As the geographical reach of Body Control Pilates has grown as a result of international publishing deals on the various books and on Lynne's videos, so we have started to build teaching and support activities in parts of the world as varied as North America, Australia, Portugal and Spain.

Underpinning this rapid expansion, our prime focus has continued to be the development of teaching skills and knowledge, and ensuring that everyone working within the Body Control Pilates 'family' has access to the latest knowledge with regard to relevant research and techniques, and, last but not least, that the numerous benefits of Pilates remain accessible to as wide a segment of the population as possible through our network of teachers and through the books and videos.

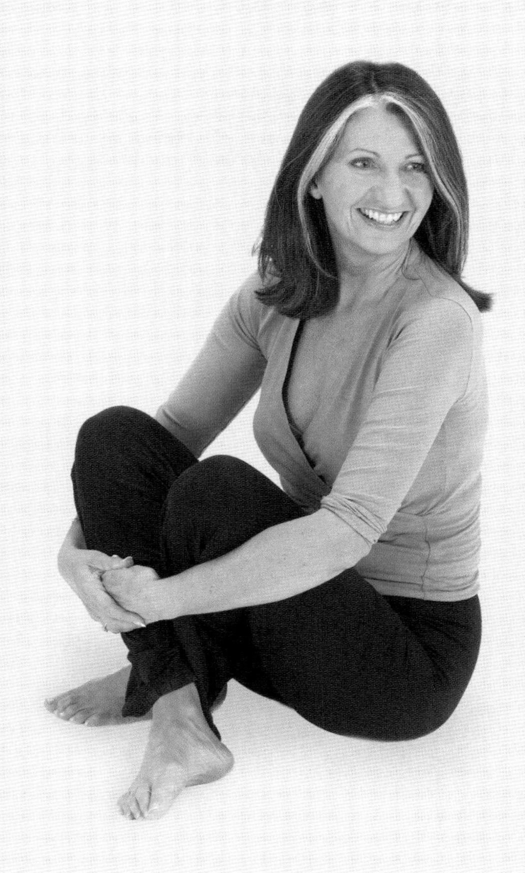

3 The Pregnancy Programme: How to Use this Book

Everyone should read the introductory chapters before starting the programme and pay particular attention to 'When Is It Not Safe to Exercise?' on pages 22–3. The programme is then divided into the following chapters:

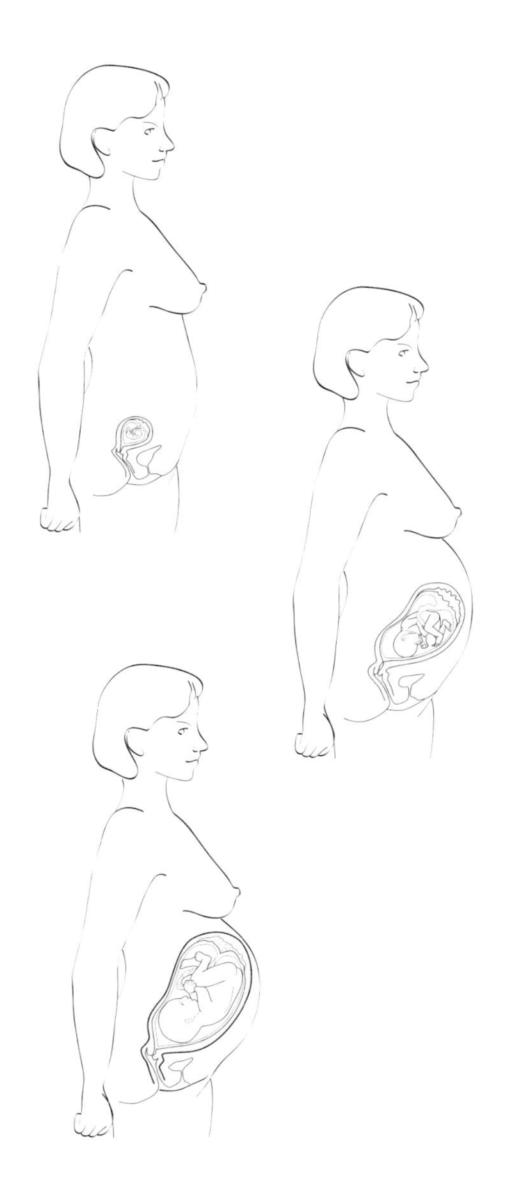

The Basics of Body Control Pilates

– Breathing. Alignment. Pilates Core Strength (Centring).

Preparing for Your Pregnancy

– Why Prepare? Exercises. Workouts.

The First Trimester (0–12 weeks)

– What's Happening to Your Body? Taking Up Pilates. Guidelines for Exercise. Exercises. Workouts.

The Second Trimester (13–26 weeks)

– What's Happening to Your Body? Taking up Pilates. Guidelines for Exercise. Exercises. Workouts.

The Third Trimester (27–34 weeks)

– What's Happening to your Body? Getting on to and up from the Floor. Guidelines for Exercise. Exercises. Workouts.

The First 6 Weeks After the Birth

– Normal Deliveries. Pelvic Floor Exercises. Exercise Programme.

– Caesarean Births. Circulation and Breathing Exercises. Exercise Programme.

Getting Back into Shape (6 Weeks Plus)

– Normal Deliveries. The Rec Check.

– Caesarean Births.

– Workouts.

Practising Pilates before and during my pregnancy helped keep me strong, healthy and well-balanced (literally). It was an ideal way to stay fit and active when I was pregnant, and, under careful supervision, allowed me to continue to enjoy exercise and develop the strength and stamina necessary for an active birth. Since giving birth, I have returned to Pilates with pleasure, finding it both relaxing and stimulating, and it's helped me return to a (more-or-less) pre-pregnancy figure without stress. – Dr Charlotte Grant

Having experienced a sports injury and nearly twenty years of back pain and discomfort. I was overjoyed but nervous when I found out I was pregnant. I had suffered from sciatica over the years and wasn't sure how my body would cope once the hormones began to relax my muscles and ligaments or with the growing weight of the baby. I decided to try Pilates and began once I was fourteen weeks pregnant.

It was a revelation to discover I could make a difference to my posture and strength even while I was pregnant. I had two sessions a week and I was closely monitored as each month passed and my body changed. Pilates gave me something I never believed I would have again: confidence in my body. Confidence it could improve, belief I didn't have to be in pain, and the most amazing gift was the total trust that my body would complete a healthy pregnany and a natural, active birth. I knew I had the stamina, strength, self-assurance and peace of mind not to panic. The birth was a wonderful experience and a lot of this was due to what I had gained from Pilates.

My baby is now five months old. I am working towards regaining my figure, but with an internal strength and a flexibility which I never had before. I know Pilates will always be part of my life to help manage my body as I grow older, perhaps through a second pregnancy and ultimately to maintain a healthy, mobile, pain-free body. – Fiona Ratti

The exercises in this book are designed for women who are preparing for pregnancy, are having a normal pregnancy, or are post-natal with no complications. There are certain contraindications to exercise in pregnancy and we have listed these on pages 22–3. However, it is impossible to list all the contraindications, which is why you *must* visit your doctor or midwife to obtain permission to follow this programme. It is possible that your GP or midwife will be unaware of the Pilates Method. If this is the case, we recommend you take this book with you so your practitioner can get an idea of the nature of Pilates exercises.

Hopefully, you will be attending regular appointments at your antenatal clinic and **it is worth asking at each visit** if it is still all right for you to continue to exercise, because your condition may have changed.

If you have never done Pilates before you should wait until you are 16 weeks pregnant and have been given the go ahead to exercise by your practitioner. Turn to pages 37–9 for guidance on how to take up Pilates during your pregnancy.

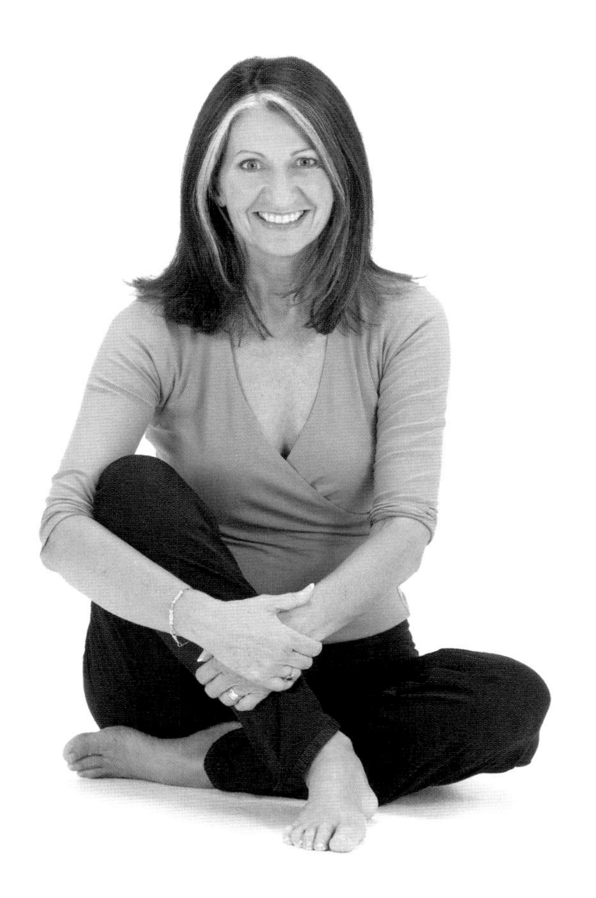

Preparing for Pregnancy

If you are planning to become pregnant and have not done Pilates before then you will need to learn the basics starting on page 44 first, and then read the chapter on Preparing for Your Pregnancy, and do the Preparatory Exercises starting on page 64. If you have done Pilates before, go straight to the chapter on Preparing for Your Pregnancy.

If You Have Done Pilates Before You Become Pregnant

Once you are pregnant, if you have followed the Preparing for Your Pregnancy programme (page 64), you may commence the first trimester exercises when your doctor or midwife has given you the all-clear. Learn the exercises given in that chapter; you can then try the different workouts at the end of the chapter. These workouts include suitable exercises that you will have already learnt in Preparing for Your Pregnancy. We have given you 5 balanced workouts to do. Most of the workouts contain 10 to 12 exercises. Ideally, you should do all 5 workouts each week. If you have more time on one day you can always do two workouts, then skip a couple of days.

If you have been attending Pilates classes – refamiliarize yourself with the Body Control Pilates approach by studying the chapter on the basics starting on page 44. You may then, providing your practitioner has given you the go-ahead, proceed with the programme for the first trimester.

Taking Up Pilates in Your Pregnancy

If you have not tried Pilates before you became pregnant, we advise you to wait until you are at least 16 weeks pregnant before you start the programme. This means you will have to learn the basics and those recommended exercises which appeared in the chapters on Preparing for Pregnancy and The First Trimester and which are now part of your workouts. Bear in mind that by 16 weeks you should avoid lying on your back for longer than 3 minutes, so change position frequently. All the other guidelines for the second trimester will also apply. A summary of the exercises you need to know if you are beginning the programme at 16 weeks follows opposite. Notice that we have excluded any exercise which is not suitable for you to do as a pregnant newcomer to Pilates.

From Chapter 5:
The Basics of Body Control Pilates

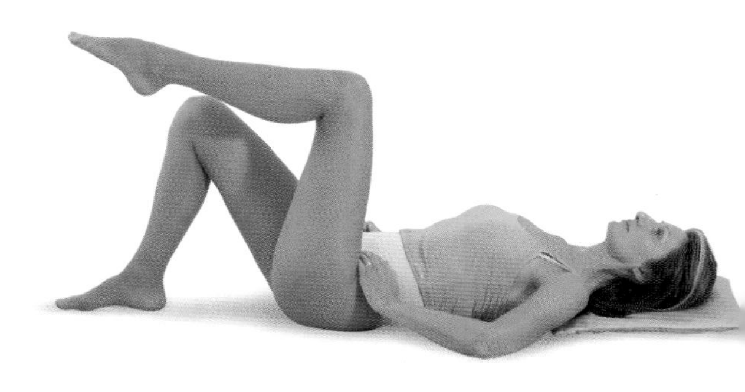

From Chapter 6:
Preparing for Your Pregnancy:

- The Full Starfish 65
- Hip Rolls (feet down) 81
- Rolling Down a Wall 84
- Sitting Side Reach 86
- Abductor Lifts 87
- Adductor Lifts 89
- The Rest Position 93

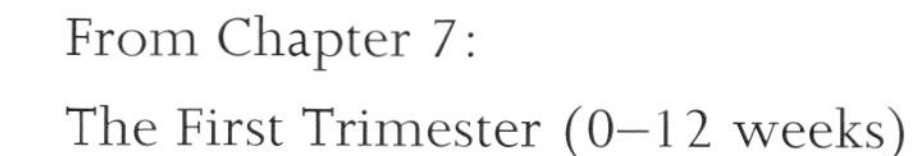

From Chapter 7:
The First Trimester (0–12 weeks)

- Demi Pliés in Turn Out 100
- The Dumb Waiter 101
- Single Leg Circles 102
- Arm Circles With and Without Weights 104
- Threading a Needle 110
- Ankle Circles 112

You are now ready to start the main programme for the second trimester.

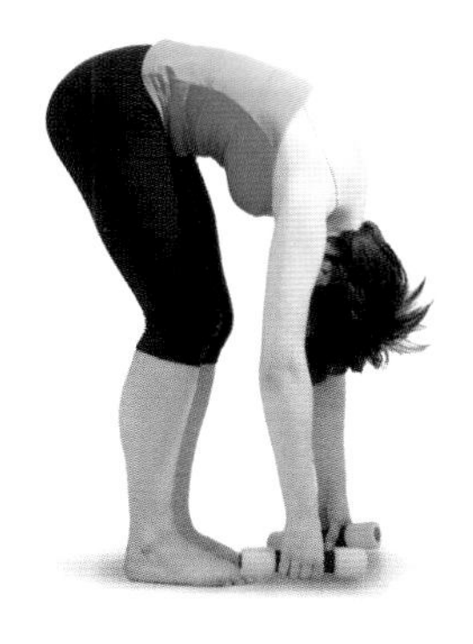

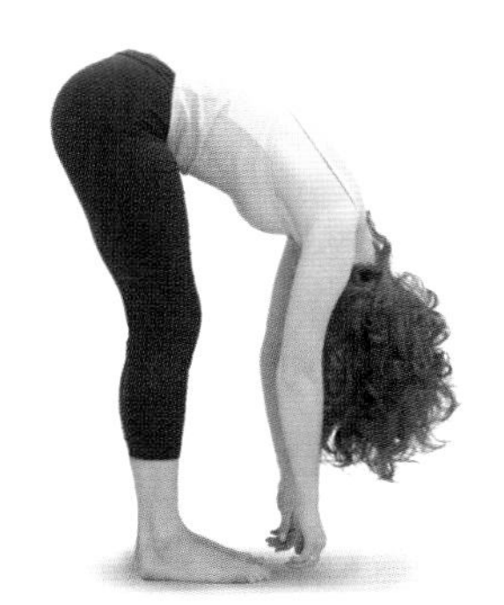

IMPORTANT NOTE

Remember to change position after each exercise so that you do not stay on your back for longer than 3 minutes. Intersperse with sitting or standing or front-lying exercises (while you can).

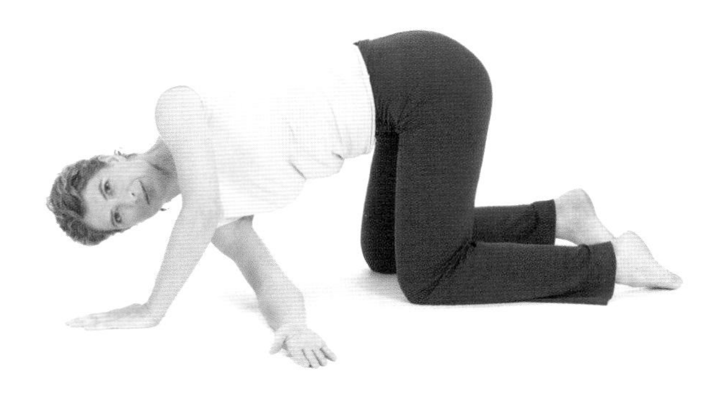

Working With a Teacher

This book has been designed as a self-help manual, but there is no doubt that it is better to work in person with a qualified Body Control Pilates teacher. Many Body Control Pilates teachers have undertaken further training in working with pregnancy and run small classes for pregnant women or offer personal training. Please avoid large, casual, drop-in classes that are not geared for pregnant women. Ideally, you will have been doing classes before you became pregnant. If this is the case and your teacher is qualified to teach pregnant women, it is usually all right to continue in a general class. The information given in this book will help you and your teacher decide which exercises are appropriate. See Further Information on page 184 to find a Body Control Pilates teacher.

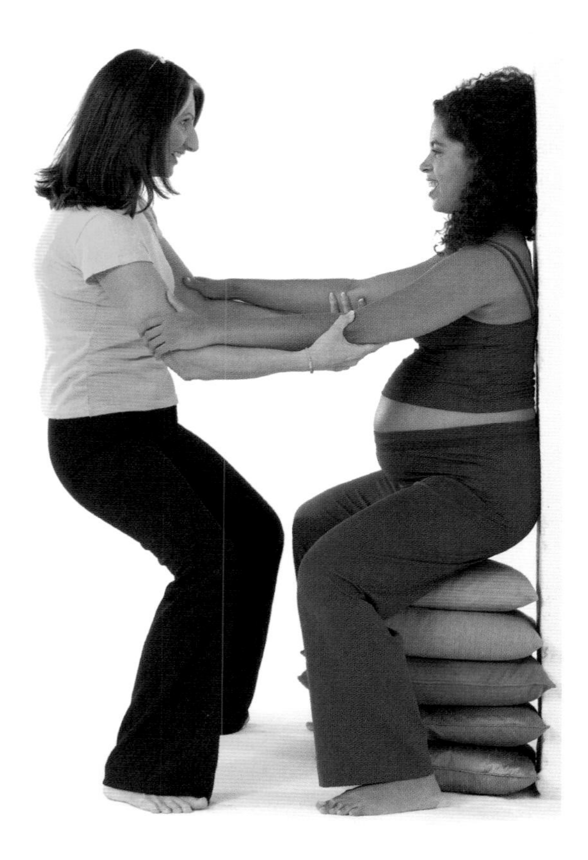

Other Advice

Cardiovascular Exercise

Cardiovascular work is very valuable and should be encouraged in normal pregnancies, but certain considerations need to be taken into account, see below. Unfortunately we cannot cover all aspects of aerobic exercise but we can offer guidelines.

Walking, cycling and swimming are highly recommended. Avoid recreational activities such as scuba diving where there is a risk of foetal decompression, contact sports (soccer, hockey) or sports that may involve a fall (horse riding, judo, gymnastics).

General Guidelines for *Aerobic Activities*

- Exercise should be regular. Aim to do 30 minutes of aerobic exercise, ideally 5 times a week. This can be accumulative – that is, for example, 3x10 minute sessions in one day. Do not tire yourself, but do stay active. Remember, a brisk walk will raise your heart rate.
- Maternal pulse rate should not exceed 150 beats per minute (individuality!).
- Wear a supportive bra.
- Your temperature should not exceed 38°C (102°F). There is a risk of damage to the baby if your temperature rises too high.
- Do not exercise with a temperature.
- Do not exercise in the heat of the day. If indoors, use a well-ventilated cool room. Similarly, do not use saunas, jacuzzis or hot tubs!
- If walking or running in the streets, avoid polluted traffic areas, and let someone know where you are going and the time when you are due back.
- Drink plenty of water.
- When exercising, the glucose levels available to the baby may be decreased and may result in a lower weight – so avoid low blood sugar. Keep the levels stable by eating complex carbohydrates, such as baked potatoes, whole grain cereals, etc., 2–3 hours before exercise.

Nutrition

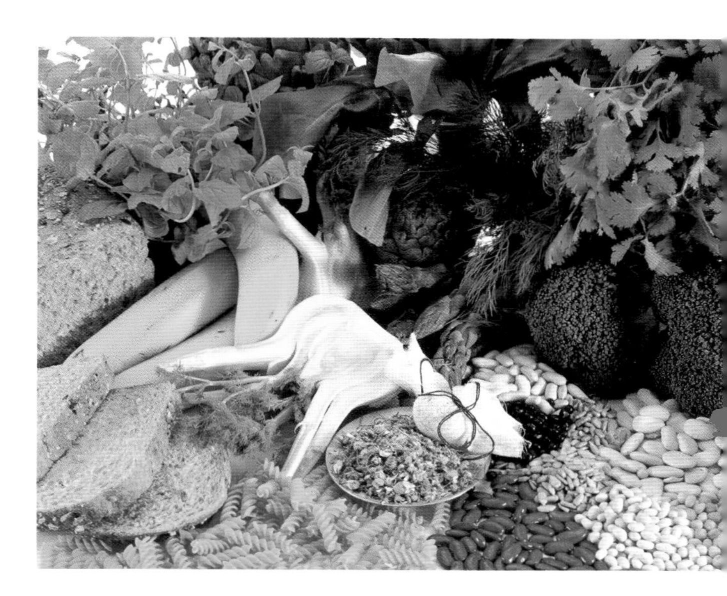

It is beyond the scope of this book to give dietary advice, but clearly a properly balanced diet will contribute to the health of mother and baby. Good nutrition for the mother will ensure appropriate blood flow, temperature and nutrition to the baby and don't forget to try to drink at least 12 glasses of water a day.

4 Before You Begin

- Make sure you have checked with your doctor or midwife that it is all right for you to exercise, and keep checking thoughout your pregnancy.
- Read pages 22–3 and 35–9 on how to use this book.
- Be sure you have no pressing unfinished business.
- Take the telephone off the hook, or put the answering machine on.
- You may prefer silence, otherwise put on some unobtrusive relaxing music.
- All exercises except standing exercises should be done on a padded mat.
- Wear something warm and comfortable, allowing free movement.
- Barefoot is best, non-slip socks otherwise.
- The best time to exercise is usually in the late afternoon or early evening when your muscles are already warmed up as a result of the day's activity. Exercising in the morning is fine, but you will need to take longer to warm up thoroughly. Be flexible, as you will probably need to adjust the timing of your session according to how you feel. It's no good trying to exercise through morning sickness or if you are feeling very tired or have indigestion.
- You need space to work in.
- Items you may need include a sturdy chair, a small, flat but firm pillow for under your head or a folded towel, several larger pillows, a long scarf or a stretchband and a tennis ball.

Please do not exercise if:

- You are feeling unwell or tired.
- You have just eaten a heavy meal.
- You have been drinking alcohol.
- You are in pain.
- You are feeling nauseous.
- You have a temperature.

- Please see contraindications on page 22 and also When to Stop Exercising on page 23.
- Some of the exercises given in the chapter on Preparing for Your Pregnancy are not suitable during pregnancy, and have therefore been left out of the recommended workouts.
- If you have a back problem, you will need to consult your medical practitioner. Many of the exercises are wonderful for back-related problems, but you should always take expert advice.

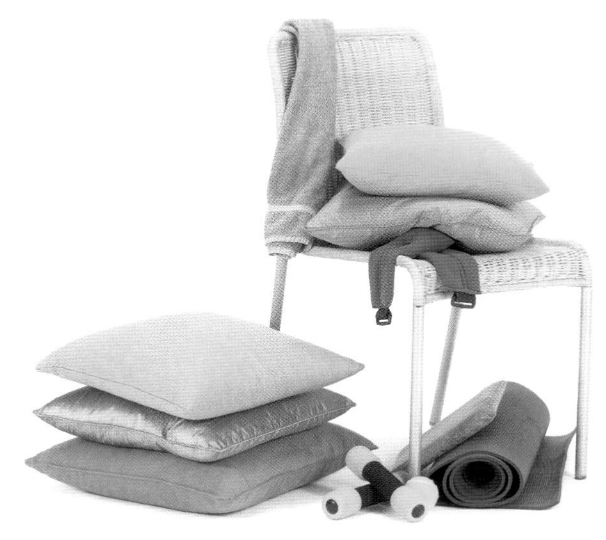

5 The Basics of Body Control Pilates

Step by step we are now going to teach you the skills you need to perform the exercises well. Once you have mastered one skill you can move on to the next. You will find that learning one skill helps with the others. Remember how you felt on your first driving lesson? There was so much to remember: steering, clutch, gears, brake, mirrors, signals, etc. Then, all of a sudden, everything fell into place and you could drive easily without having to think about it (still watching the road though!). This is because how to drive had entered your muscle memory banks, along with learning to swim, to ride a bike and so on. It's exactly the same with Pilates. At first you will despair – keeping neutral, breathing wide, zipping up and hollowing – but eventually it all comes together and you can move on.

The basic skills you need to begin are breathing, good alignment and centring.

Breathing

Stand in front of a mirror and watch as you take a deep breath. Do your shoulders rise up around the ears or does your lower stomach expand when you breathe in? Most of us breathe inefficiently. Ideally, you should breathe wide and full into your back and sides.

This type of breathing – called thoracic or lateral breathing – makes the upper body more fluid and mobile. The lungs become like bellows, with the lower ribcage expanding wide as you breathe in and closing down as you breathe out. As you breathe in your diaphragm automatically descends; the aim is not to stop this but rather to focus on the movement making it widthways and into the back. The lungs are just like balloons and they need to expand in all directions as they fill with air. Unfortunately for most of us the balloons never get to be fully inflated! Learning how to breathe thoracically will change that.

Try this simple exercise:

- Sit or stand tall (you will never be able to breathe well unless you lengthen up through the body because bad posture compresses your ribcage). Wrap a scarf or a towel around your ribs, crossing it over at the front.

- Holding the opposite ends of the scarf and pulling it tight gently, breathe in and allow your ribs to expand the scarf (watch that you do not lift the breastbone too high).

- As you breathe out, you may gently squeeze the scarf to help fully empty your lungs and relax the ribcage, allowing the breastbone to soften.

Breathing out, you will also engage the pelvic floor and hollow the abdomen (explained in Centring: Pilates Core Strength on page 48) to give both lumbar and pelvic stability as you move. Ultimately you will need to keep these muscles engaged as you breathe in and out.

Also important to Pilates is the timing of the breath. Most people find this difficult at first, especially if you are used to other fitness regimes, but once you have mastered it, it makes sense. As a general rule:

- Breathe in to prepare for a movement.

- Breathe out fully, zipping up and hollowing (see page 49) and move.

- Breathe in, still zipped and hollowed, to recover.

When you are pregnant you are more prone to feeling dizzy, so make sure you do not overbreathe. Your breathing should be at a natural, easy pace. If you need to take an extra breath or change the timing of the breath, please do so. Never, ever, hold your breath.

Moving on the exhalation enables you to relax into the movement and prevents you from tensing. It also offers greater core stability at the hardest part of the exercise and safeguards against holding the breath, which can unduly stress the heart and lead to serious complications.

Remember to focus on the out-breath completely, emptying the lungs. When you do this, the in-breath will naturally come flooding in.

As your pregnancy progresses and your uterus grows, the lower ribs will flare, making lateral breathing quite difficult. It is perfectly fine at this time to allow your breathing to be more apical, that is higher and shallower, do not force lateral breathing at this late stage – go with the natural flow.

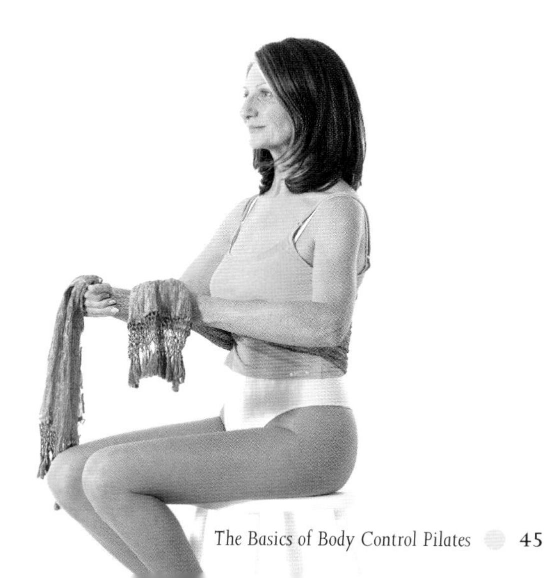

Alignment

We have discussed at length the importance of good alignment on page 11. Use the Relaxation Position (page 26) and Standing Well (page 16) and Sitting Well (page 17) to remind yourself how to position the body correctly. The following exercise will help you to find your neutral pelvis and spinal positions.

IMPORTANT NOTE

You should not stay in this position for longer than 3 minutes in your second and third trimesters.

The Compass: Finding Neutral

In Pilates, the aim is to have the pelvis and spine in their natural, neutral positions. The angle of your pelvis affects the angle of your spine. Learning how to find your neutral pelvis is the first step towards finding your neutral spinal position.

- Lie in the Relaxation Position (page 26).
- Imagine you have a compass on your lower abdomen. Your navel is north and your pubic bone south, with west and east on either side. Now we'll try two incorrect positions in order to find the correct one.
- Tilt your pelvis up towards north. The pelvis will tuck under, the waist will flatten and the curve of the lower back is lost as your tailbone lifts off the mat. You will also shorten the muscles around your hips and abdominals.
- Next, carefully and gently move the pelvis in the other direction so that it tilts down towards south. Don't go too far, just a little way. (Avoid this bit if you have a back injury.) The low back arches, the ribs flare and the stomach sticks out. Come back to the starting position.
- Aim for a neutral position between these two extremes. Go back to the image of the compass and think of the pointer as a spirit level. When you are in neutral, the pubic and pelvic bones will be level north/south and east/west. Your sacrum will rest squarely on the mat. You should feel as though the tailbone is lengthening away along the mat. Try also to keep both sides of the waist long and equal.
- Now bring your awareness to your spine. Think of the 'S' shape of the spine. Think of lengthening through the spine while keeping those natural curves.

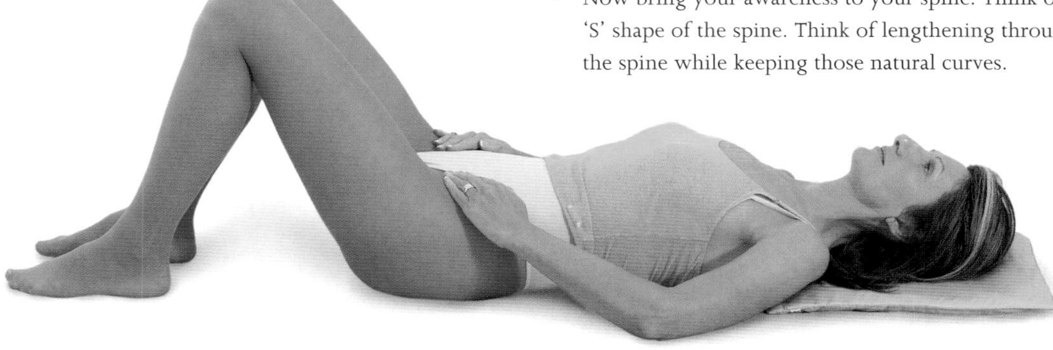

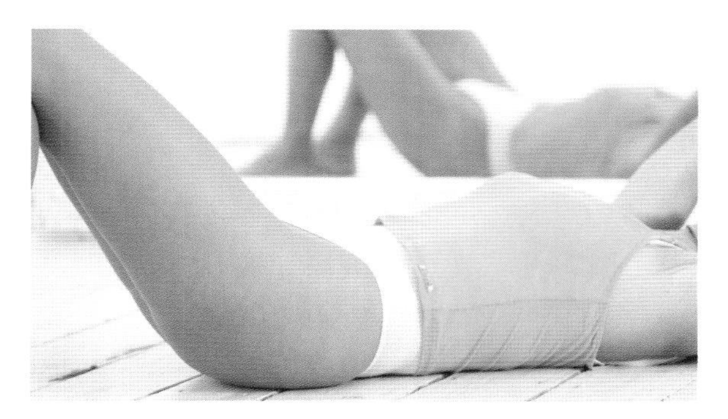

North

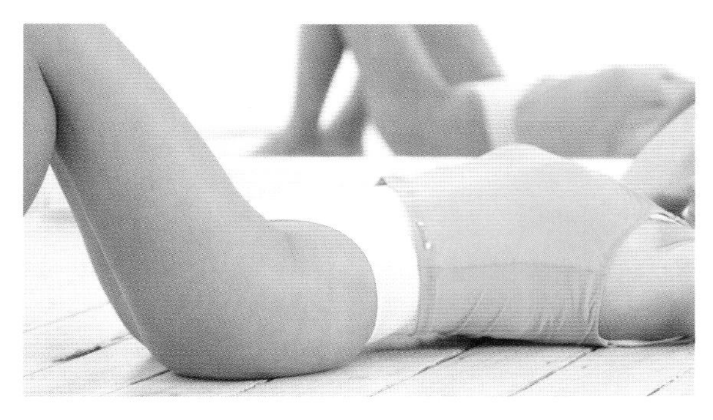

South

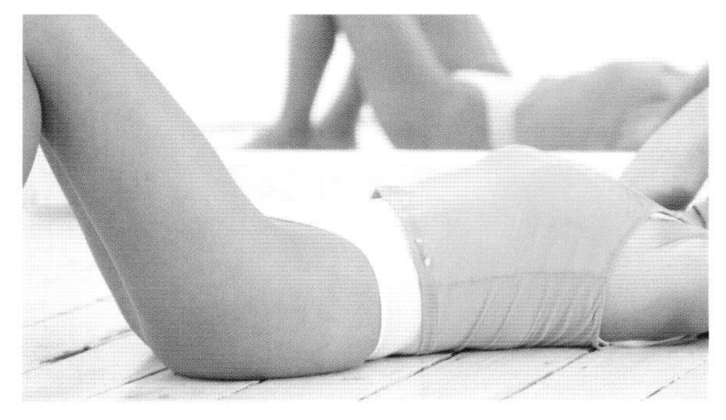

Neutral

Once you are familiar with this position in the Relaxation Position, you should practise finding neutral while standing, sitting and lying on your side so that it becomes normal. Please note that if the muscles around the pelvis are very out of balance, you may find neutral difficult to maintain. When this is the case, consult your practitioner, as it is often necessary to work in what is the best neutral you can achieve, or to use support in the way of towels or flat pillows. Usually after a few months, as the muscles begin to rebalance, neutral becomes more comfortable.

I loved the strength Pilates gave my body to cope with pregnancy, birth and breastfeeding – twice!

– Sally Hemeon

Centring: Pilates Core Strength

Now we need to locate and engage those all-important core stabilizing muscles. One of the most important aspects in all stability work is engaging the muscles at the right amount. Muscles can work from 0–100 per cent effort. Try standing up and tightening your buttocks as much as you can (100 per cent). Now try to release them about 50 per cent. Then, let go half as much again to 25 per cent – that's how much you should be working your deep muscles. This is because these muscles have to work for you all day, every day. If you work them harder they will become fatigued, when they need endurance. For basic stability work we want you to work the muscles gently at no more than 25 per cent. Of course, when you are doing an advanced exercise such as The Hundred (page 78) you will need to work a bit harder to stay stable. The key is to engage them gently to begin with and then gradually increase their recruitment.

Back to the pelvic floor. Where are your pelvic floor muscles? They are the muscles which run from the front to the back of the base of the trunk forming a sling on which all your abdominal contents rest! For our exercises we will be needing to isolate only parts of your pelvic floor and to do so in a particular way. Be warned, this isn't easy and requires a lot of patience, a lot of practice and a lot of concentration!

We are trying to engage the muscles of the vagina and the urethra. One way to help locate these muscles is to suck your thumb as you draw them up inside. It sounds crazy, but it's effective! You want to think about these muscles as if you are lifting up from behind (as if to prevent passing wind, but without clenching the buttocks!). The muscles lift up from back to front and, as they lift up and forwards, they also draw together side to side (see the Pelvic Elevator opposite) – think of a camera shutter closing!

Try this exercise for awareness of where you are working and how hard you should work.

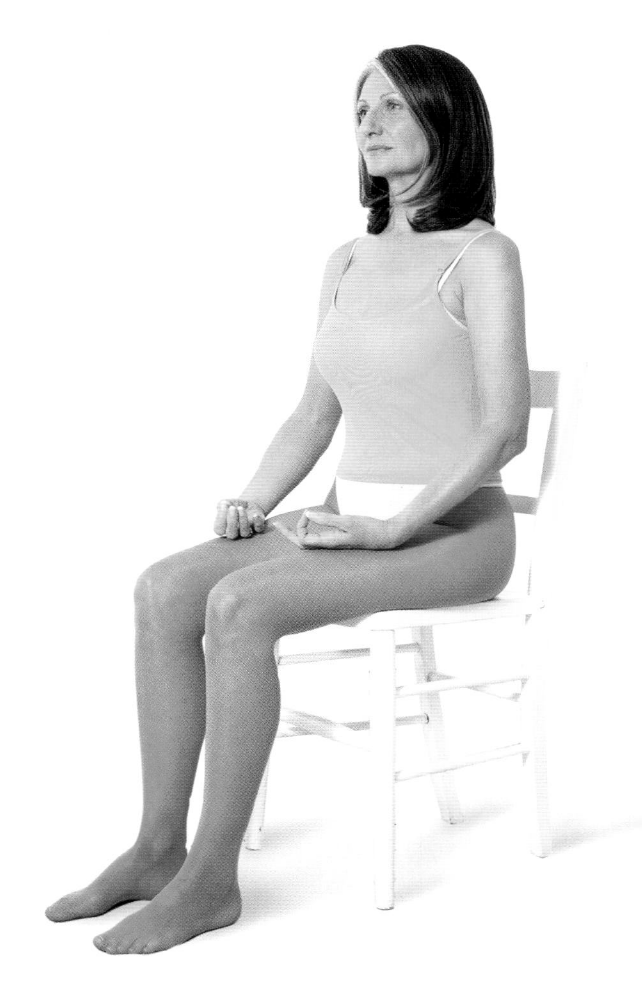

The Pelvic Elevator (sitting)

Aim

This exercise was created to isolate and engage the deep stabilizing muscles of the pelvis, pelvic floor and spine – transversus abdominis and multifidus. The idea is to use the pelvic floor muscles to help engage them. We will be doing the same exercise later in the programme to strengthen the pelvic floor.

Equipment

A sturdy chair.

Starting Position

Sit tall on an upright chair making sure you are sitting square, with the weight even on both buttocks. Imagine your pelvic floor is like the lift in a building and this exercise requires you to take the lift up to the first floor. Later on we will teach you to take the lift higher.

Action

1. Breathe in wide and full into your back and sides, lengthening up through the spine.
2. As you breathe out, draw up the muscles of your pelvic floor as if you are trying to prevent the flow of water. Draw the muscles together from back to front, lifting them forwards and up. Take the pelvic lift up to the first floor of the building to about the level of your bladder, well below the navel. This is as far as you need to engage the muscles for zip up and hollow.
3. Breathe in and release the lift back to the ground floor.

Watchpoints

- When you reached the first floor, you should have felt the deep lower abdominals engage. This is transversus abdominis coming into play. By starting the action from underneath, you encourage the six-pack muscle, rectus abdominis, to stay quiet. If you were to take the lift all the way to the top floor, you would probably be engaging the muscles at over 30 per cent and the six pack would take over. Sometimes you may have to zip up to the second floor, but still keep the action low and gentle.
- Do not allow the buttock muscles to join in.
- Keep your jaw relaxed.
- Don't take your shoulders up to the top floor too – keep them down and relaxed.
- Try not to grip around your hips.
- Keep the pelvis and spine quite still.
- Think of bringing your sitting bones together.

Once you have found your pelvic floor muscles, learn how to engage them in different positions. When you have found them, it should be easier to isolate transversus abdominis. To engage these muscles correctly (at no more than 25 per cent) think of:

- hollowing
- scooping
- drawing back the abdominals towards the spine
- sucking in

As your uterus grows and you get bigger, you may find the image of 'hollowing' a difficult one to conceive! But the action should remain the same even though there will not be much in the way of actual hollowing going on. You can also think of lifting your bump.

The instruction from now on will be to 'zip up and hollow' – you need to imagine you have an internal zip that goes from your pelvic floor up, and to hollow the lower abdominals back to the spine. Remember, to the first floor only! Keep the action low and gentle. As your uterus grows it may be more helpful to think of **'zip and lift'** rather than 'zip up and hollow'.

The following three positions will help ensure this is done correctly:

Stabilizing on all Fours

Try this wearing just your underwear, with a mirror underneath you. You can check to see if your six pack remains quiet!

Starting Position

Kneel on all fours; hands beneath your shoulders and knees beneath your hips. Keep your elbows soft and directed backwards (this helps keep your shoulder blades down). Have the top of your head lengthening away from your tailbone and your pelvis in neutral. Imagine a small pool of water resting on the base of your spine (it will help you to find neutral).

Action

1. Breathe in wide to prepare.
2. Breathe out and zip up and hollow the lower abdominals in towards the spine. Your back should not move; the pool of water stays put.
3. Breathe in and release.
4. Now try again, only this time add your lateral thoracic breathing – staying zipped while breathing in and out.

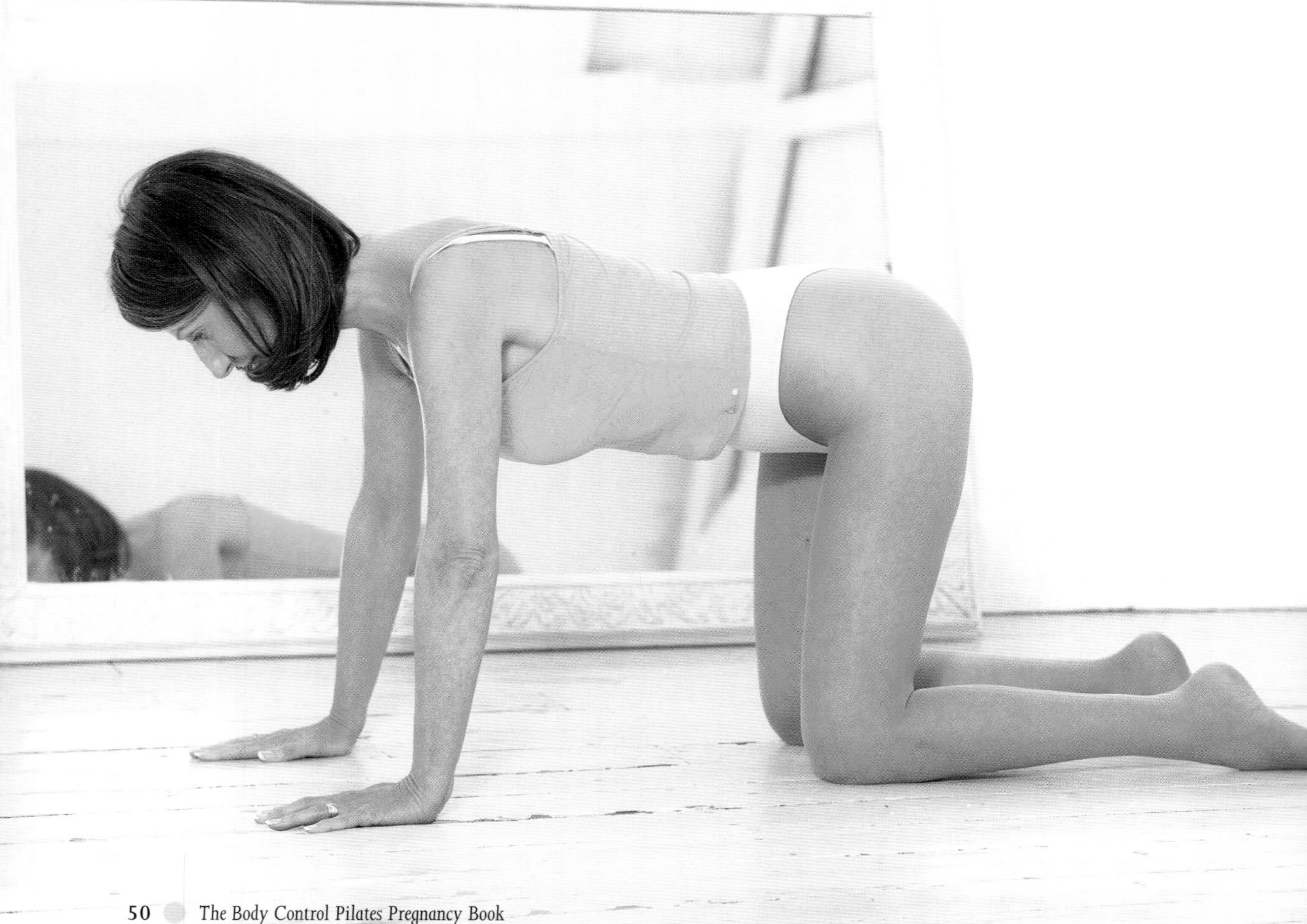

Stabilizing in Prone Lying

Try this position if you can still lie on your front.

Equipment
A flat, firm cushion.

Starting Position
Lie face down, resting your head on your folded hands. Open the shoulders out and relax the upper back (use a small, flat cushion under your abdomen if your low back is uncomfortable). Your legs are shoulder-distance apart and relaxed.

Action
1. Breathe in wide to prepare.
2. Breathe out, zip up from the pelvic floor and hollow the lower abdominals back to your spine away from the floor.
3. Imagine there is a small precious egg just above the pubic bone that must not be crushed. Do not tighten the buttocks – there should be no movement in the pelvis or the spine.
4. Now try to stay zipped as you breath in and out.

This then, is your strong centre. For most of the exercises, you will be asked to zip up and hollow, before and during your movements.

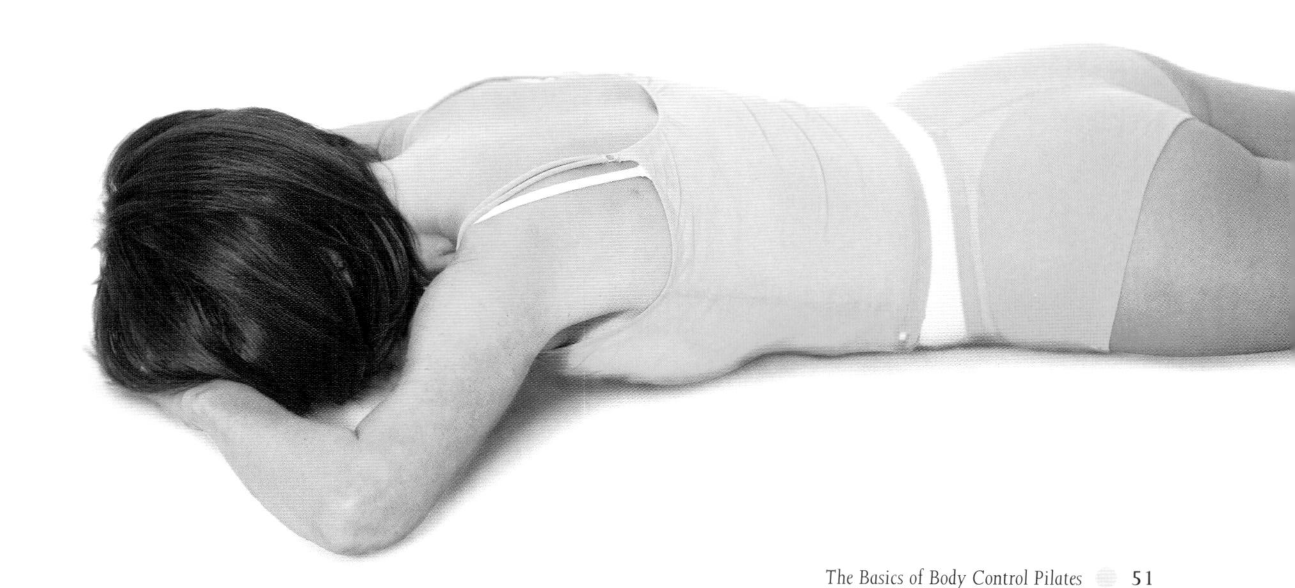

Stabilizing in the Relaxation Position

Starting Position

Lie in the Relaxation Position and go through your checklist (page 26). Find your hip bones (they are where your hipster jeans would, or used to, sit). Place your fingers an inch inwards and downwards from these bones and feel the lower abdominals are relaxed.

Action

1. Breathe in wide to prepare, and lengthen through the spine.
2. Breathe out and zip up and hollow. Your fingers should feel your abdominals engage. Breathe normally as you keep these muscles working – try to think of them sinking back towards the spine. If they bulk up or go very tight you are working too hard.
3. Work up to keeping zipped for 5 breaths. Do not hold your breath.

Watchpoints

- Check constantly that you are still breathing! And that your ribcage is moving.
- Do not allow the pelvis to tuck under – stay neutral with your pelvis level.
- Do not push into the spine. Keep your tailbone on the floor and lengthening away.

NOTE

As your bump grows you can think of 'zip and lift the bump' rather than 'zip and hollow'.

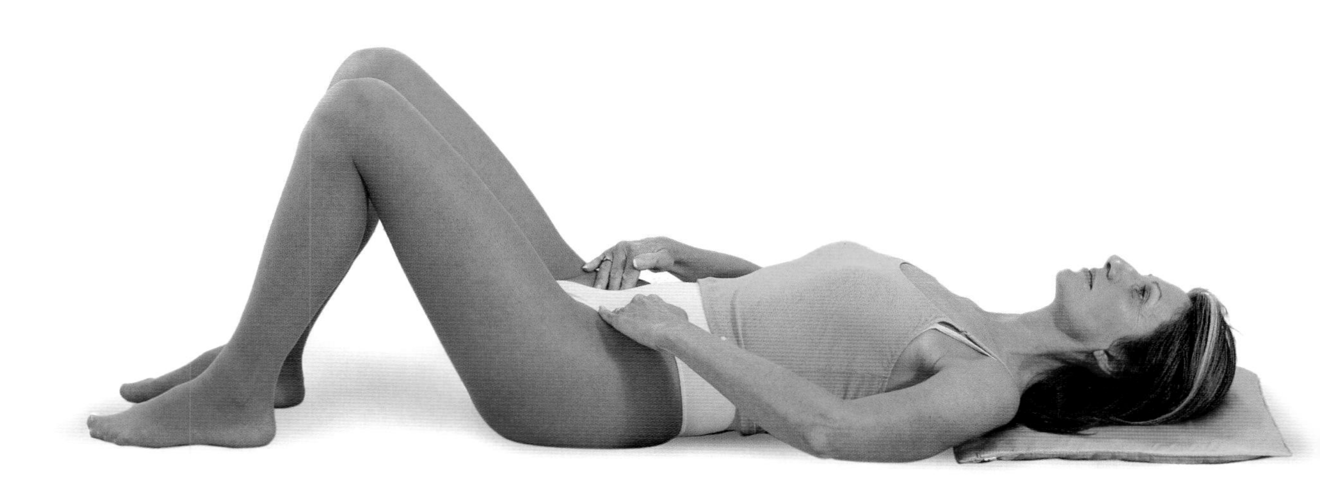

Stabilizing in Side-lying

This is a useful position in which to practise stability in your second and third trimesters.

Equipment
Three cushions.

Starting Position
Lie on your left side in a straight line. Have your underneath arm stretched out in a line with your body and place a flat cushion between your ear and the arm so that your neck keeps in line with your spine. Place shoulder over shoulder, hip over hip. Have your knees together, one directly over the other, bent just less than 90° angle. You can place a small cushion between them to help keep your pelvis in a good position. If you like, you can put a cushion under your bump to support you. If viewed from the air, you will look like you are sitting on a chair.

Action
1. Breathe in wide and full and lengthen through the body.
2. Breathe out and zip up and hollow.
3. Stay zipped while you breathe normally for about 5 breaths. Do not allow your waist to sink into the floor. Keep lengthening through the body.

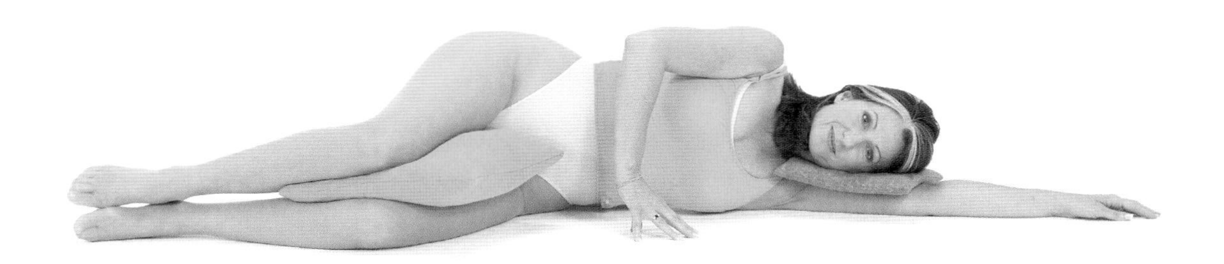

Pelvic Stability: Leg Slides, Knee Drops, Knee Folds and Turn Out

Aim

Having mastered breathing, correct alignment and the creation of a strong centre, you must learn how to add movement co-ordinating all this. It isn't easy to begin with, but soon becomes automatic. Meanwhile, the process of learning this co-ordination is fabulous mental and physical training as it stimulates that two-way communication between the brain and the muscles.

Start with small movements, then build up to more complicated combinations. Below are four movements to practise, all of them requiring you to keep the pelvis completely still. It is useful to imagine that you have a set of car headlamps on your pelvis, shining at the ceiling. The beam should be fixed, not mimicking searchlights! You can vary which exercises you practise in each session, but the Starting Position is the same for all three.

Starting Position

Adopt the Relaxation Position (page 26). Check that your pelvis is in neutral, tailbone down and lengthening away, then place your hands on your hip bones to check for unwanted movement.

Action for Leg Slides

- Breathe in wide and full to prepare.
- Breathe out and zip up and hollow.
- Sliding one leg away along the floor in line with your hips, keep the lower abdominals engaged and the pelvis still, stable and in neutral.
- Breathe in to your lower ribcage while you return the leg to the bent position, trying to keep the pelvic bones still. If you cannot yet breathe in and maintain a strong centre, take an extra breath and return the leg on the out-breath.
- Repeat 5 times with each leg.

IMPORTANT NOTE

During your second and third trimesters you will need to change position after 3 minutes – try stabilizing in Side-lying described on page 53.

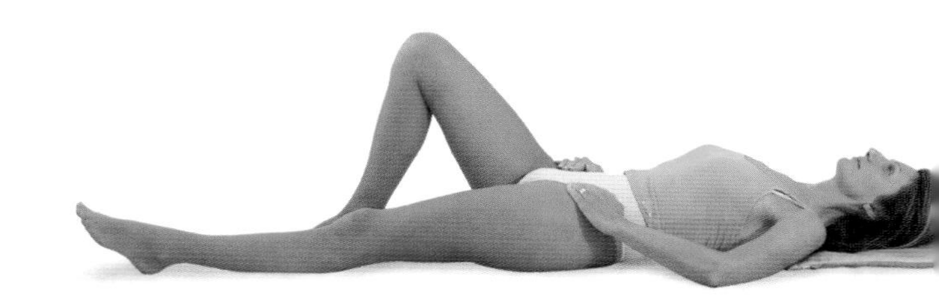

Leg Slides

Action for Knee Drops

1. Breathe in wide and full to prepare.
2. Breathe out, zip up and hollow, and allow one knee to open slowly to the side. Go only as far as the pelvis can stay still. It will want to roll from side to side – don't let it.
3. Breathe in, still zipped and hollowed, as the knee returns to the centre.
4. Repeat 5 times with each leg.

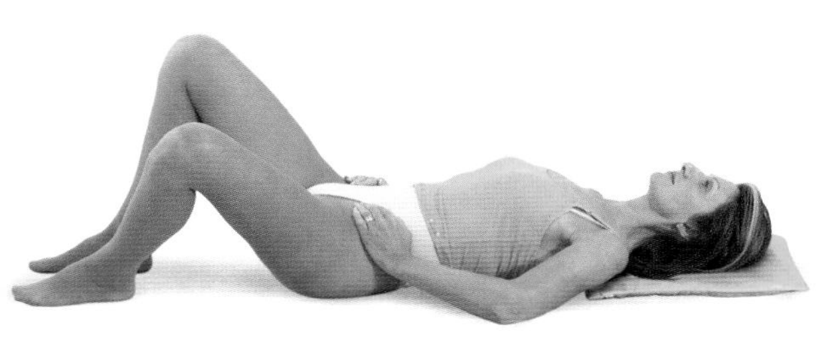

Knee Drops

Action for Knee Folds

With this movement it is particularly useful to feel that the muscles stay 'scooped' and do not bulge while you fold the knee in. Very gently feel the muscles engage as you zip up and hollow.

1. Breathe in wide and full to prepare.
2. Breathe out and zip up and hollow, then fold the right knee up. Think of the thigh bone dropping down into the hip and anchoring there.
3. Do not lose your neutral pelvis – the tailbone stays down – and do not rely on the other leg to stabilize you. Imagine your foot is on a cream doughnut and you don't want to press down on it.
4. Breathe in and hold.
5. Breathe out, still zipped and hollowed, as you slowly return the foot to the floor.
6. Repeat up to 5 times with each leg.

If you find this very difficult you can bring your feet closer to you.

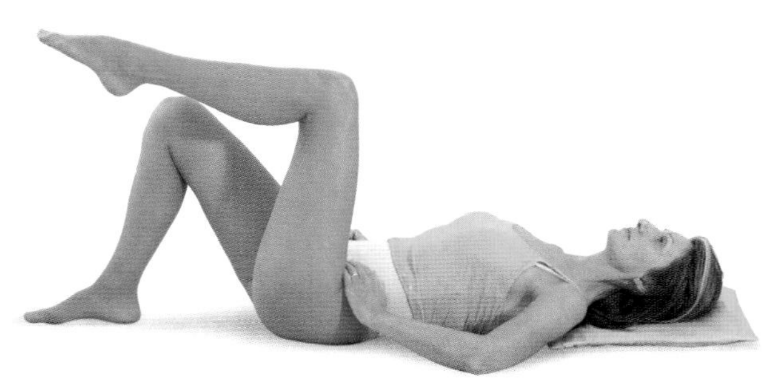

Knee Folds

Action for Turn Out

This next movement involves turning the leg out from the hip and is a preparation for exercises such as the Star (page 105) where the legs are held in a turned-out position. It works the deep gluteal muscles, especially gluteus medius, which is one of the main stabilizing muscles of the pelvis.

1. Breathe in wide and full to prepare.
2. Breathe out, zip up and hollow, then fold the right knee up. Think of the thigh bone dropping down into the hip and anchoring there.
3. Breathe out, zip up and hollow, then turn the right leg out from the hip bringing the foot to touch the left knee, if possible. Keep the knee in line with the hip.
4. Do not allow the pelvis to tilt or twist or turn, keep it central and stable – headlamps glued to the ceiling!
5. Breathe in and then out and zip up and hollow as you reverse the movement to return the foot to the floor.
6. Repeat 5 times to each side.

Watchpoints

- Remember you are trying to avoid even the slightest movement of the pelvis. It helps to think of the waist being long and even on both sides as you make the movement.
- Try to keep your neck and jaw released throughout.

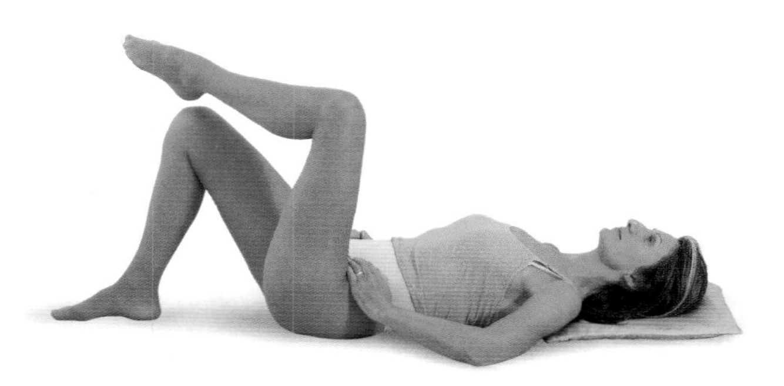

Turnout

Scapular Stability

The final part of our girdle of strength concerns the muscles of the mid-back, which set the shoulder blades down into the back. These are the lower trapezius and the serratus anterior muscles. When they are working correctly they stabilize the scapulae, placing them and the shoulder joint itself in the best position to allow for good mechanics. As your breasts grow, there is a natural tendency to stoop. Our exercises are designed to open out the chest, teach good alignment of the head, neck and shoulders and strengthen the stabilizing muscles. The idea is to re-educate your movement so that when you reach up with your arms the action is free-flowing and natural.

To find these muscles, try this exercise:

NOTE

Please take advice if you suffer from sciatica

Shoulder Reach

The goal of this exercise is be aware of the muscles in the mid-back that connect the shoulder blades down into the back.

IMPORTANT NOTE

During your second and third trimesters you will need to change position after 3 minutes.

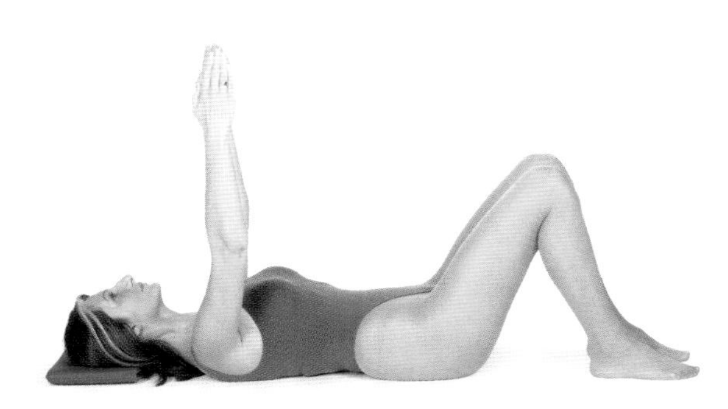

Starting Position

Lie in the Relaxation Position (page 26). Have your arms resting down by your sides with your palms on the floor.

Action

1. Breathe in wide to prepare, and lengthen through the spine.
2. Breathe out, zip up and hollow, and slide your arms down towards your feet, reaching through the fingertips and turning your palms to face inwards. As you do so you will feel your shoulder blades connecting down into your back and your upper body will open out.
3. Breathe in and hold the stretch; be aware of the distance between your ears and your shoulders.
4. Breathe out and relax.
5. Repeat up to 5 times.

Moving on

1. Follow directions 1–3 above then breathe out and, still reaching through your fingers, raise both arms until they are directly above your shoulders. As you do so, keep your upper shoulders soft and your elbows open.
2. Breathe in and lower.
3. Repeat up to 5 times.

Watchpoints

- There is a tendency for the ribcage to flare up; keep the ribcage calm and down.
- Your neck should remain soft and released; the back of the neck stays long.

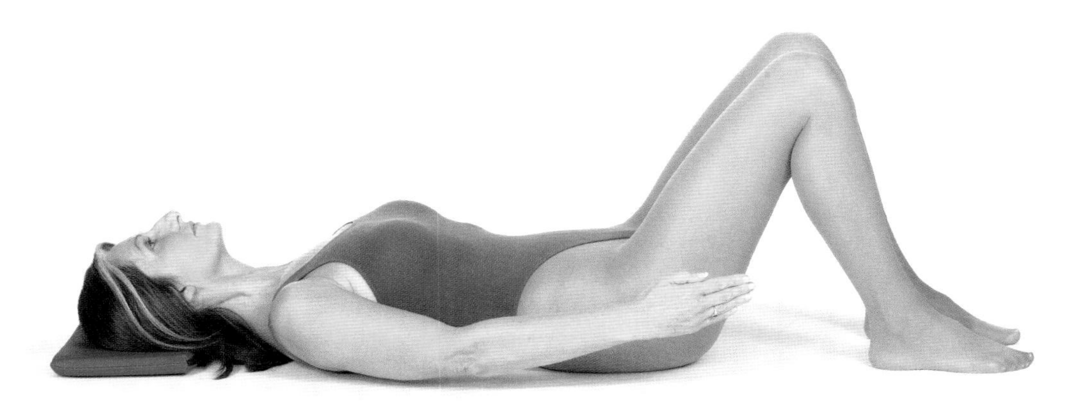

The Dart (Stage One)

In this exercise we are going to find the same muscles, but lying face down. You can continue to exercise lying on your front for as long as is comfortable.

Equipment
A flat cushion (optional).

Starting Position
Lie face down (you can place a flat cushion under your forehead to allow you to breathe) with your arms by your sides and your palms facing your body. Your neck is long. Your legs are relaxed but in parallel.

Action
1. Breathe in to prepare and lengthen through the spine, tucking your chin in gently as if you were holding a ripe peach beneath it.
2. Breathe out, zip up and hollow, and slide your shoulder blades down into your back, lengthening your fingers down towards your feet.
3. The top of your head stays lengthening away from you too.
4. Keep looking straight down at the floor. Do not tip your head back.
5. Breathe in, and feel the length of your body from the tips of your toes to the top of your head.
6. Breathe out, still zipping, and release.

Watchpoints
- Keep hollowing the lower abdominals.
- Do not strain the neck – it should feel released as your shoulders engage down into your back. Think of a swan's neck growing out between its wings.
- Keep your feet on the floor.
- Stop if you feel at all uncomfortable in the low back. This exercise can also be done with the feet hip-width apart and the thigh and buttock muscles relaxed.

Moving on . . . the muscles that you felt pulling your shoulder blades down into your back are the stabilizing muscles. Now that you have located them, try to feel them working in this next exercise.

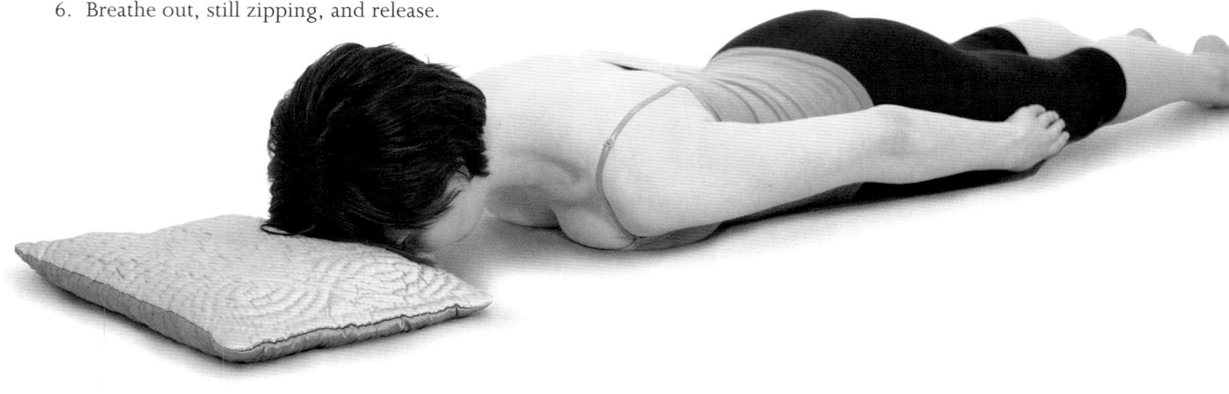

Floating Arms

We all have a tendency to overuse the upper part of our shoulders (the upper trapezius). As you raise your arm, think of this order of movement:

- first, just your arm moves up and out
- then you feel the shoulder blade start to move – it coils down and around the back of the ribcage
- finally, the collarbone (clavicle) rises up

With good movement, the shoulder blade will move in the same way as the ballast on a security barrier would move.

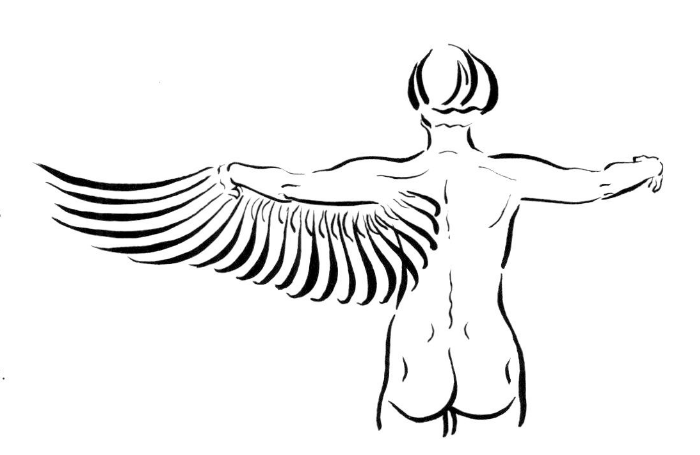

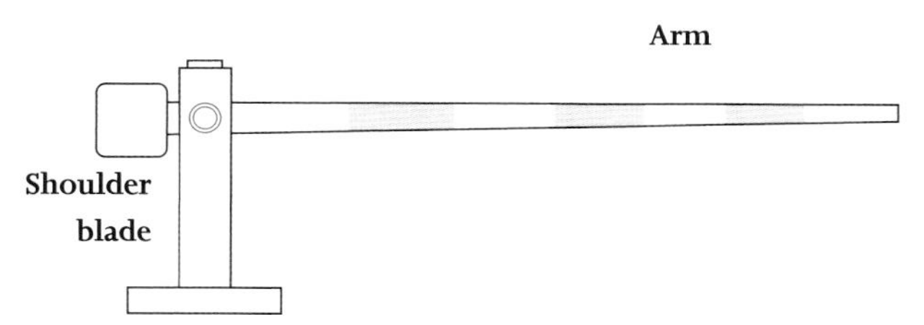

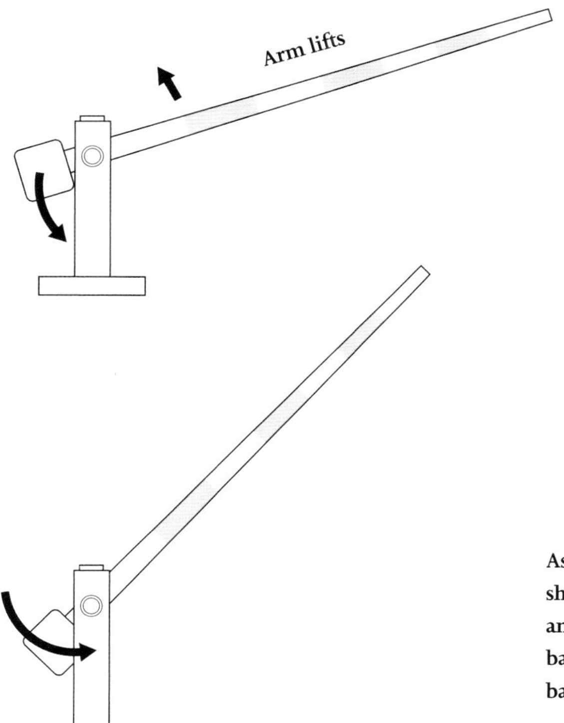

As your arm rises, your shoulder blade drops down and around the ribcage like the ballast moves as the security barrier (your arm) lifts.

Starting Position

Stand or sit tall. Place your left hand on your right shoulder. Feel your collar bone; you are going to try to keep the collar bone still for the first part of the movement. Your hand can check that the upper part of your shoulder remains 'quiet' for as long as possible. Very often this part overworks, so think of it staying soft and released, while the lower trapezius below your shoulder blades work to set the shoulder blades down into your back.

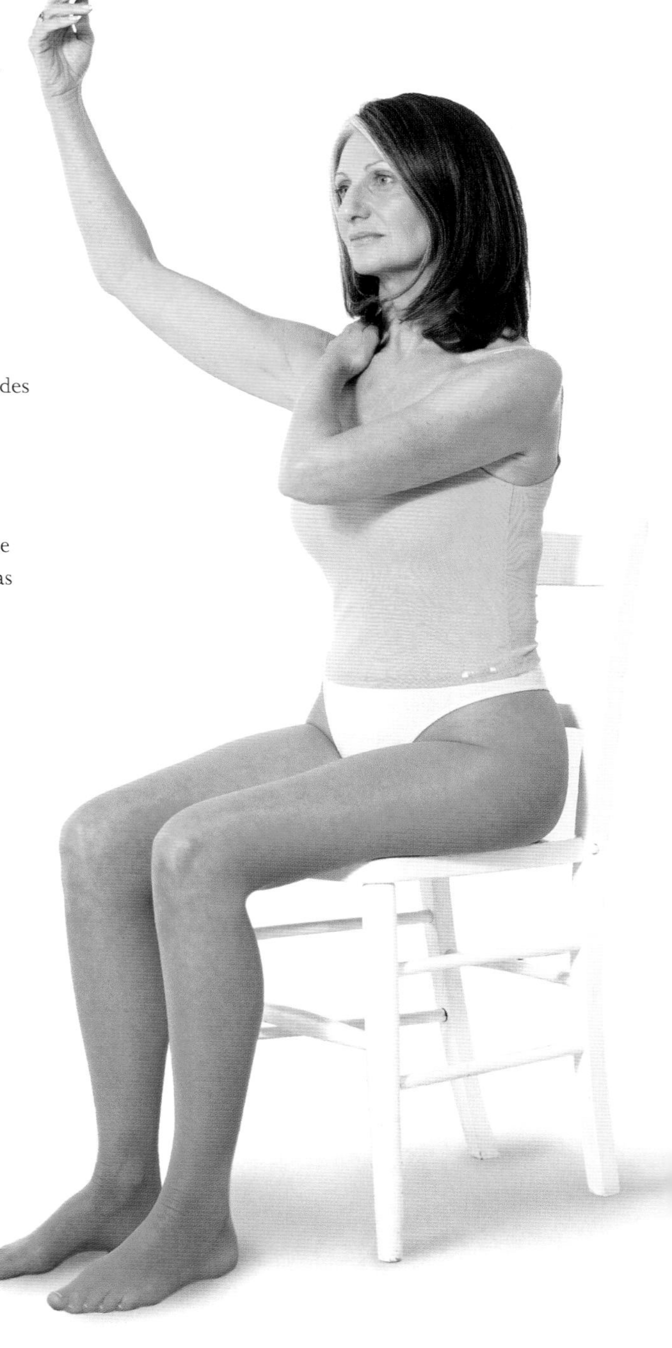

Action

1. Breathe in to prepare and lengthen up through the spine, letting the neck relax.
2. Breathe out and zip up and hollow. Slowly begin to raise the arm, reaching wide out of the shoulder blades like a bird's wing. Think of the hand as leading the arm: the arm follows the hand as it floats upwards.
3. Rotate the arm so that the palm opens to the ceiling as the arm reaches shoulder level. Try to keep the shoulder under your hand as still as possible, and the shoulder blades dropping down into your back for as long as possible.
4. Breathe in as you lower the arms to your side.
5. Repeat 3 times with each arm.

Watchpoints

- Keep a sense of openness in the upper body.
- Do not allow your upper body to shift to the side, keep centred.
- Think of the security barrier image on the previous page.

The Starfish (arms only)

Aim

To learn good upper-body movement.

As your arm moves back think of what you learnt in Floating Arms (page 59). Focus on keeping the upper shoulders relaxed and the ribcage down.

IMPORTANT NOTE

You will need to change position regularly every 3 minutes if you are in your last two trimesters.

Starting Position

Lie in the Relaxation Position (page 26) with your arms down by your sides.

Action

1. Breathe in wide into your lower ribcage to prepare.
2. Breathe out, zip up and hollow, and start to take one arm back as if to touch the floor. You may not be able to touch it comfortably, so only move the arm as far back as you can.
3. Do not force the arm – keep it soft and open, with the elbow bent. Think of the shoulder blade setting down into your back. **The ribs stay calm and down**. Do not allow the back to arch at all.
4. Breathe in as you return the arm to your side.
5. Repeat 5 times with each arm.

Watchpoints

- Keep your neck released.
- Don't bring the arm too close to your head.
- Try to keep the action smooth and flowing.

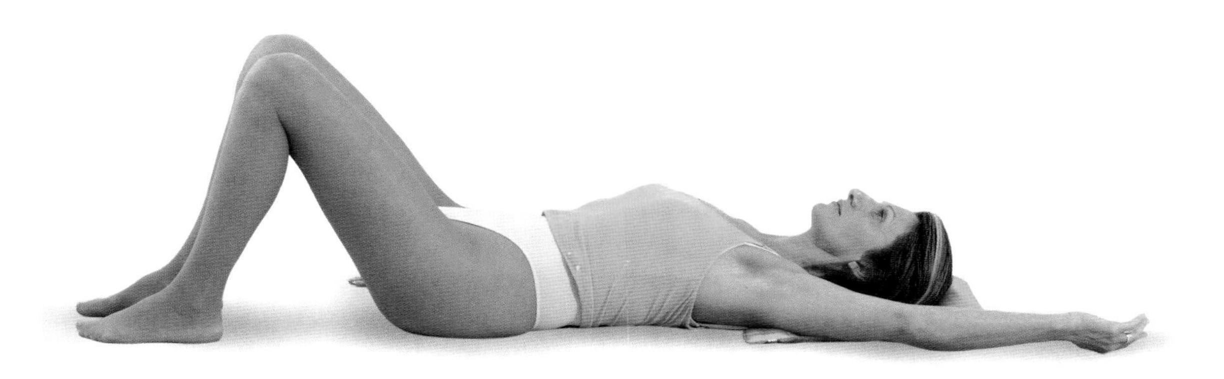

Neck Rolls and Chin Tucks

This is the final exercise in this basic skills section, which will help you correctly position your head on your neck. You will be using this 'nod' when you perform many of the exercises in the main programme.

An important aspect in re-educating the head–neck relationship lies in the relative strength of the neck extensors (which tilt the head back) and the flexors (which tilt the head forward). If you think about the body positioned at a desk or a steering wheel, the head is usually thrust forward and tipped back – a muscle imbalance. By relaxing the jaw, lengthening the back of the neck and gently tucking the chin in, this balance can be redressed.

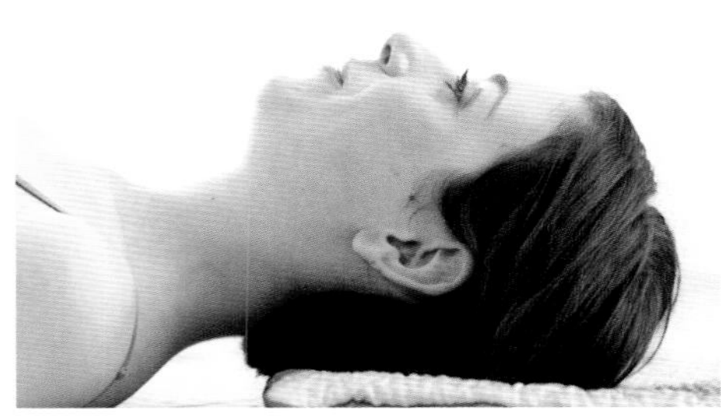

Starting position

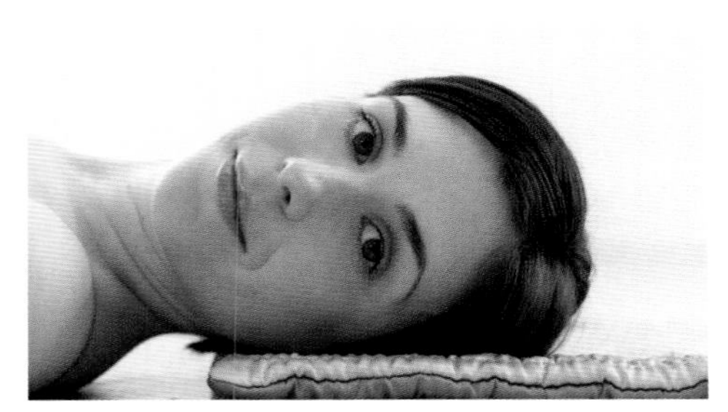

Neck Rolls

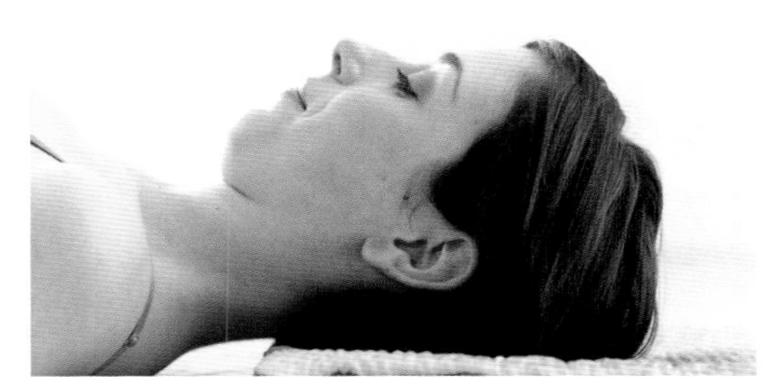

Chin Tucks

Aim

This exercise releases tension from the neck, freeing the cervical spine. It also uses the deep stabilizers of the neck, and lengthens the neck extensors.

Please note that this is a subtle movement – you should tuck your chin in gently. It is a nodding action.

Starting Position

Lie in the Relaxation Position (page 26) with your arms resting on your lower abdomen. Only use a flat pillow for this exercise if you are uncomfortable without one because your head rolls better if you do not use one.

Action

1. Release your neck and jaw, allowing your tongue to widen at its base. Keep the neck nicely lengthened and soften your breastbone. Allow the shoulder blades to widen and melt into the floor.
2. Now, allow your head to roll slowly to one side.
3. Bring it back to the centre and over to the other side, taking your time.
4. When the neck feels free, bring the head to the centre and gently tuck your chin in, as if holding a ripe peach under it (you do not want to crush the delicate skin). Keep the head on the floor and lengthen out of the back of the neck.
5. Return the head to the centre.
6. Repeat the rolling to the side and the chin tuck 5 times.

Watchpoints

- Do not force the head or neck – just let them roll naturally.
- Do not lift the head off the floor when you tuck the chin in.

6 Preparing for Your Pregnancy

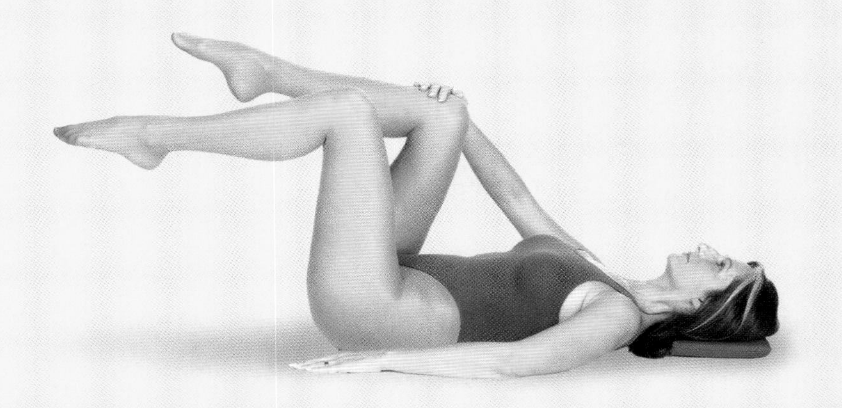

Why Prepare?

There is no doubt that the sooner you can start to do Pilates in preparation for your pregnancy the better. Pilates is not a quick-fix programme. It takes time for your body to take on board all the principles of Pilates and to remember all the correct patterns of movement. In the same way that you have to practise a tennis serve or a golf swing again and again before it becomes automatic, so you have to repeat a movement something like 10,000 times before it becomes ingrained (a muscle memory).

The Pilates Method is not just a set of exercises, it is a movement technique that teaches you to move well. It is only when you have absorbed all its principles, when you have learnt to be body aware, to breathe efficiently, to stabilize your spine, pelvis and shoulder blades, to align your body well, to move with minimum effort and maximum grace, that you will really feel the wonderful benefits that Pilates can offer. But this takes time – so the sooner you can start the programme the better.

If you have already been pregnant you will realize how many ways your body changes in a very short period of time. The fitter and healthier you are before you fall pregnant, the better you will be able to cope with those changes. For example, if you make your inner core, your deep abdominals, strong, then you will be able to carry the extra weight of the baby so much more easily and you are less likely to suffer from diastasis recti after the birth. As your uterus grows, your abdominal muscles must lengthen and the linea alba, which divides the rectus abdominis (six pack), separates to allow for this growth. If your abdominal muscles are strong before you become pregnant, this separation is not a problem and the two sides will join together again after the birth. But if your abdominal muscles are weak there is a chance that they will remain separated. If the gap remains more than 2 centimetres wide, this can be a problem.

If you are conscious of what is good and bad posture, then you are far less likely to have back and joint problems during your pregnancy. Remember, too, that all your body's systems – lymphatic, respiratory, digestive, circulatory and reproductive – will function more efficiently if you exercise regularly. So the sooner you get started the fitter you will be.

Preparatory Exercises

The Full Starfish

Aim

To combine everything you have learnt so far! To practise free-flowing movement away from a strong centre. As your arm moves back think of what you learnt in Floating Arms (page 59). As the leg slides away, think of what you learnt in Leg Slides (page 54). And, of course, don't forget your girdle of strength.

Not everyone can touch the floor behind them with their arm without arching the upper back, so do not strain. It is better to keep the ribs down than force the arm.

IMPORTANT NOTE

You will need to change position regularly every 3 minutes if you are in your last two trimesters.

Starting Position

Lie in the Relaxation Position (page 26), with your arms down by your sides.

Action

1. Breathe in wide and full to prepare.
2. Breathe out and zip up and hollow. Slide the left leg away along the floor in a line with your hips, while simultaneously taking the right arm above you in a backstroke movement. Do not allow the ribcage to lift – it stays down. Keep the pelvis completely neutral, stable and still and the stomach muscles engaged.
3. Breathe in, still zipped and hollowed, and return the limbs to the Starting Position.
4. Repeat 5 times alternating arms and legs.

Watchpoints

- Do not be tempted to overreach – the girdle of strength must stay in place.
- The pelvis stays in neutral, it is level north/south and east/west. Both sides of the waist stay even.
- Keep a sense of width and openness in the upper body and shoulders and think of the shoulder blades setting down into your back.

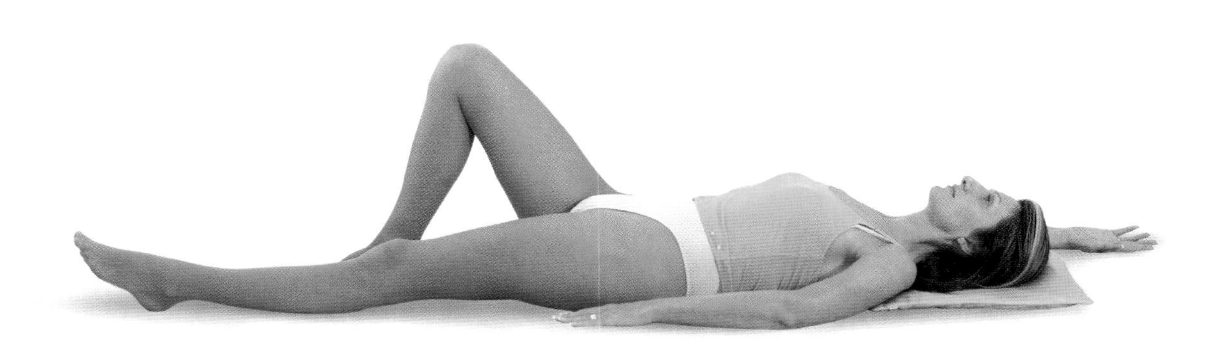

Shoulder Drops and Cross Over Shoulder Drops

A wonderful exercise that allows you to let go of any tension around the shoulders and neck. Great to do at the end of a stress-filled day.

Aim
To release tension in the upper body.

Shoulder Drop Starting Position
Lie in the Relaxation Position (page 26).

Action
1. Raise both arms towards the ceiling directly above your shoulders with the palms facing each other.
2. Reach for the ceiling with one arm, stretching through the fingertips. The shoulder blade comes off the floor. Drop the shoulder back down on to the floor.
3. Repeat up to 10 times with each arm. Feel your upper back widening and the tension in your shoulders releasing down into the floor.

Moving on . . . when you are comfortable with the above, try the following variation. You will need to keep the pelvis stable for this version, which means adding the zip up and hollow.

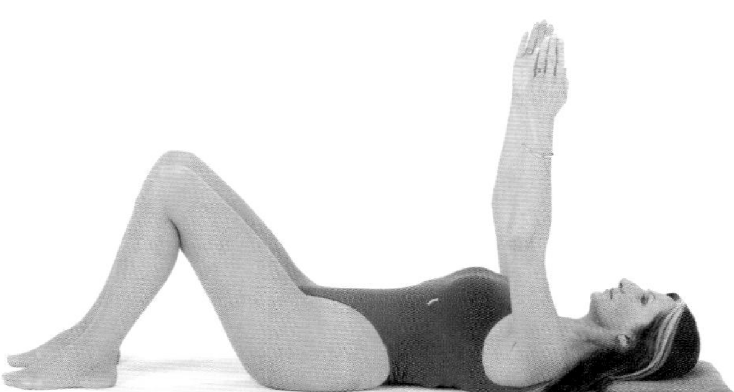

Cross Over Starting Position
Lie in the Relaxation Position (page 26).

Action
1. Breathe in wide and full to prepare.
2. Breathe out and zip up and hollow, keeping the pelvis still and square. Reach one hand up across to the other, in the direction of where the ceiling meets the wall. Your shoulder blade will leave the floor, your head should move gently with you. Enjoy the stretch between the shoulder blades.
3. Breathe in and hold the stretch.
4. Breathe out and relax the shoulder back down to the floor.
5. Repeat 10 times to each side, making sure that the pelvis stays quite still.

Watchpoints
- Whichever version you are doing, keep the distance between your ears and your shoulders.
- Do not control the shoulder as it drops, release it on to the floor.

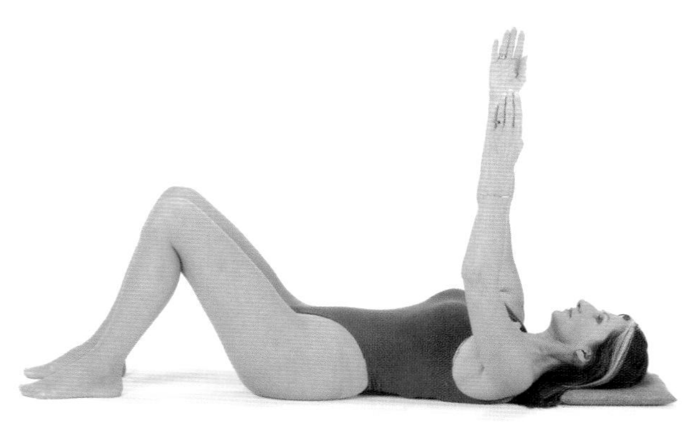

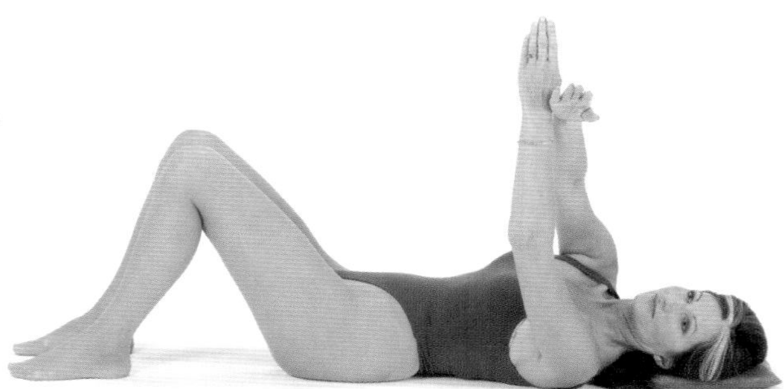

Spine Curls with Pillow Squeeze

Aim

This wonderful exercise works on the mobility of the spine. Joseph Pilates always referred to using the spine 'like a wheel', and encouraged his clients to peel their vertebra from the floor bone by bone. The good news is that it also works the buttocks and the inner thighs.

Equipment

A plump cushion.

Starting Position

Lie in the Relaxation Position (page 26), checking that your feet are in parallel but several centimetres apart, and about 30 centimetres (12 inches) away from your buttocks. Place the pillow between your knees. Your arms are relaxed down by your sides, palms facing down.

Action

1. Breathe in wide to prepare.
2. Breathe out, zip up and hollow and stay zipped throughout. Squeeze the cushion between the knees, gently engage your buttocks and curl the tailbone off the floor just a little.
3. Breathe in, and slowly curl back down to neutral, lengthening out the spine.
4. Breathe out and peel a little more of the spine off the floor. Really try to get the base of the spine open.
5. Breathe in and then breathe out as you place the spine back down, bone by bone.
6. Continue to curl more of the spine off the floor each time you go up on the exhalation. Inhale while you are raised, and exhale as you wheel the spine, vertebra by vertebra, back down on to the floor. Aim to lengthen the spine as you wheel back down. The deep abdominals and the pelvic floor stay engaged throughout and you keep squeezing the cushion between the knees.
7. Do not come up any higher than your shoulder blades. Do 5 full curls before you relax.

Watchpoints

- You must not arch the back. Keep in your mind the image of a whippet who has just been scolded, and has his tail (your tailbone) curled between his legs!
- Keep the weight even on both feet and try not to let them roll in or out.
- Keep your neck long and soft.

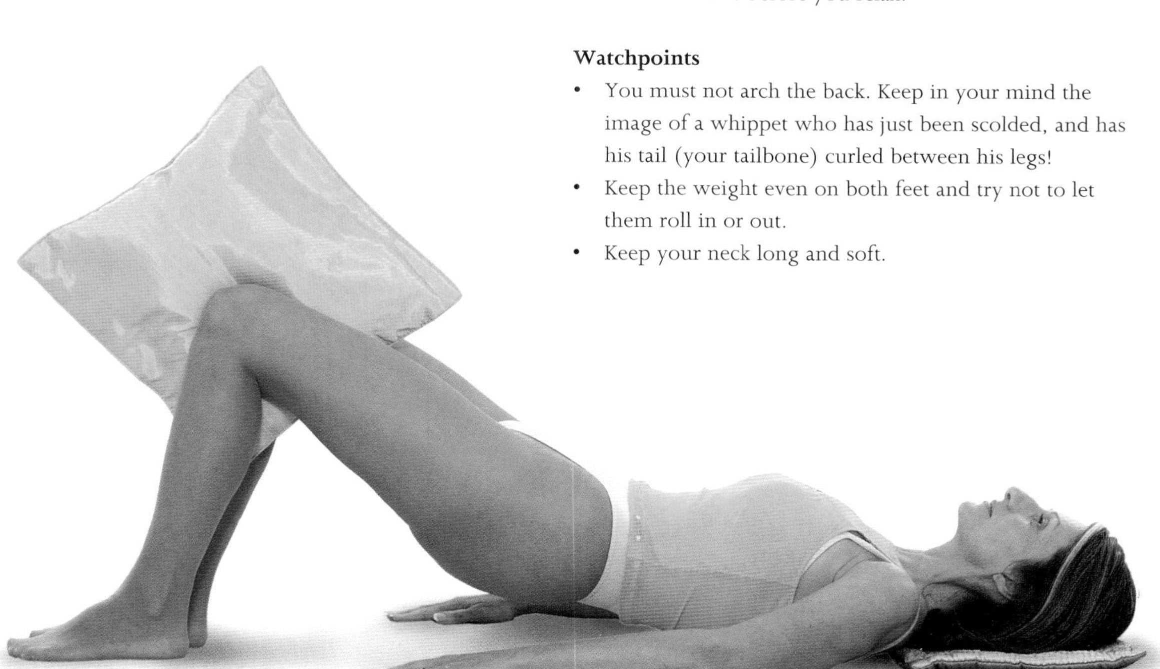

Curl Ups

Just look at the number of Watchpoints for an exercise that you have probably seen done in every gym in the country! The reason our version works so well is that you are required to pay close attention to maintaining neutral and keeping your lower abdominals hollow. This ensures that transversus abdominis stays engaged and that you are targeting the right abdominals to achieve the ultimate flat stomach. If you lose neutral, let your abdominals bulge, or fling yourself up quickly, you lose the effectiveness of the exercise and that flat stomach will remain a dream.

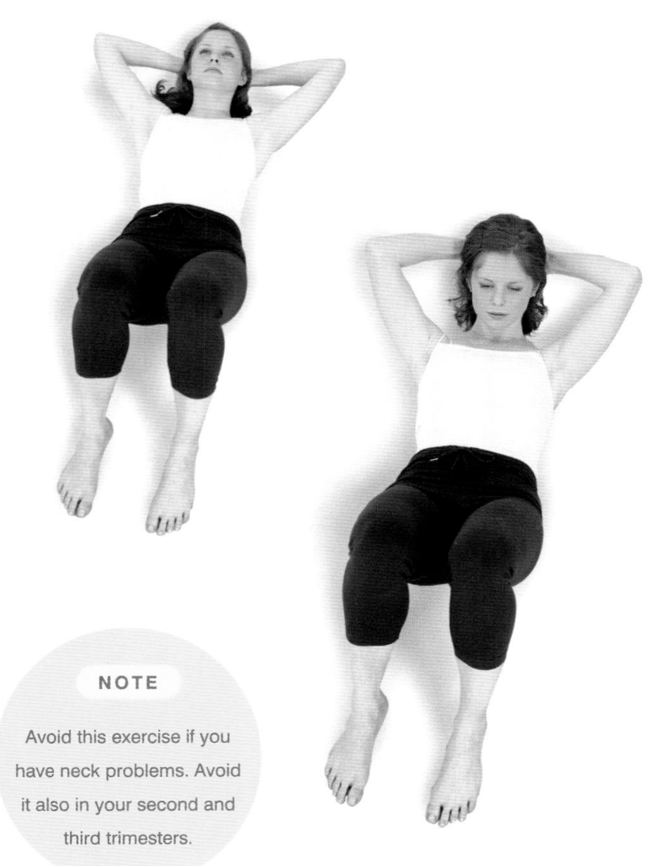

NOTE

Avoid this exercise if you have neck problems. Avoid it also in your second and third trimesters.

Aim

To strengthen the abdominals, engaging them in the correct order and with the trunk in perfect alignment.

Starting Position

Lie in the Relaxation Position (page 26). Gently release your neck by rolling the head slowly from side to side. Lightly clasp your hands behind your head to cradle and support it (at no point should you pull on your neck). Keep your elbows open just in front of your ears throughout.

Action

1. Breathe in, wide and full, to prepare.
2. Breathe out, zip up and hollow, soften your breastbone, tuck your chin in a little (as if holding a ripe peach) and curl up, breaking from the breastbone and closing the ribcage down. Your stomach must not pop up. Keep the pelvis level and the tailbone down on the floor lengthening away.
3. Breathe in and slowly curl back down, controlling the movement.
4. Repeat 10 times.

Watchpoints

- Try not to grip around the hips; keep those muscles soft.
- Stay in neutral, tailbone down on the floor and lengthening away. The front of the body keeps its length. A useful image is that there is a strip of sticky tape along the front of the body, which should not wrinkle!
- Think of peeling the upper spine, bone by bone, from the floor.
- Think of the ribs funnelling down towards the waist.
- Keep the chin gently tucked in; this is the cervical nod action you learnt in Neck Rolls (page 62), which should help keep your neck released.
- Don't close your elbows as you come up – keep them open, but within your peripheral vision.

Oblique Curl Ups

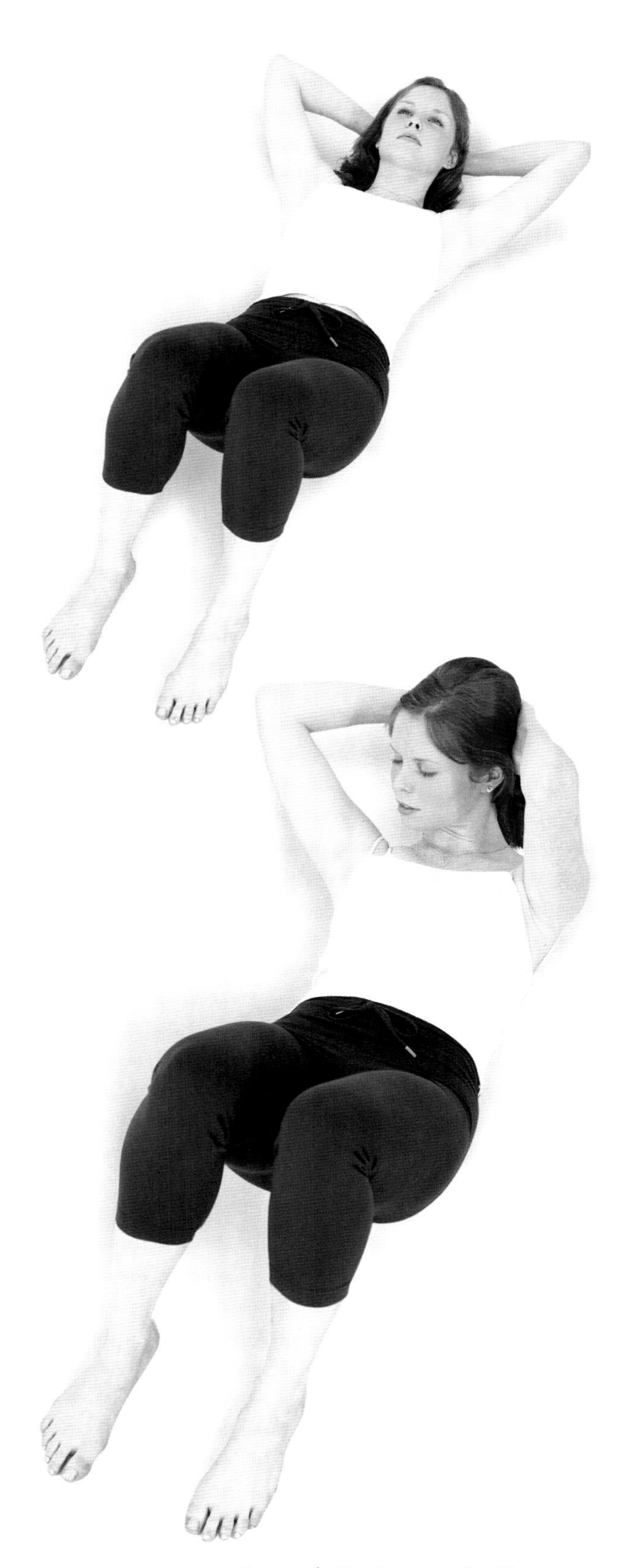

Aim

To work the obliques which wrap around your waist.

Starting Position

Lie in the Relaxation Position (page 26). Your hands are lightly clasped behind your head and your chin is gently tucked in as for Curl Ups.

Action

1. Breathe in wide and full to prepare.
2. Breathe out and zip up and hollow. Curl your upper body up, bringing your left shoulder across towards your right knee. The right elbow stays back. Your stomach must stay hollow, the pelvis stays still, square and stable.
3. Breathe in, still zipped, and slowly lower with control.
4. Repeat 5 times to each side.

Watchpoints

- The same watchpoints as for Curl Ups apply.
- Keep both sides of equal length. There is always a tendency with this exercise to shorten one side of the waist as you come up. Keep the action simple; you are going across at an oblique angle.
- Keep the upper body open, elbows back but in view.
- Focus on keeping the pelvis very still. You may find that the opposite hip wants to come up; stay square and neutral.

NOTE

Avoid this exercise if you have neck problems. Avoid it also in your second and third trimesters.

The Pelvic Elevator (sitting)

It's never too early to start these exercises because these muscles are going to be very important. Try to focus on drawing up every muscle fibre – it is the quality of the contraction that counts. Never hold your breath while contracting the pelvic floor. Try to do your pelvic floor exercises regularly throughout the day – while waiting at traffic lights, while queuing and so on.

NOTE

Pelvic floor exercises are best done in frequent batches of about 6 contractions at a time.

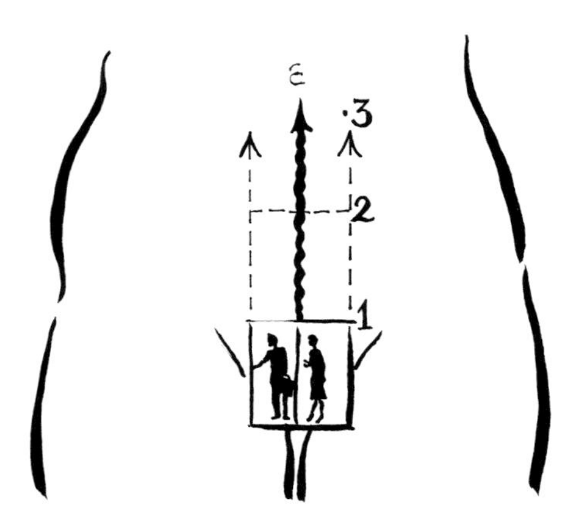

The pelvic elevator

Aim

This time we are going to use this exercise as a pelvic floor workout rather than as a way of activating transversus abdominis, which means we are going all the way up to the top floor!

Starting Position

Sit tall on an upright chair; make sure you are sitting square with the weight even on both buttocks. Imagine your pelvic floor is like the lift in a building and this exercise requires you to take the lift up to different floors of the building. There are four floors.

Action

1. Breathe in wide and full to your back and sides, then lengthen up through the spine.
2. As you breathe out, draw up the muscles of your pelvic floor as if you are trying to prevent the flow of water. Remember to draw them together from back to front, lifting forwards and up. Take the pelvic lift up to the first floor of the building.
3. Breathe in and release the lift back to the ground floor.
4. Breathe out and take the lift up to the second floor.
5. Breathe in and release.
6. Breathe out and take the lift up to the third floor.
7. Breathe in and release.
8. Now breathe out and take the lift all the way to the penthouse!
9. Breathe in and release.
10. Repeat 6 times.

Watchpoints

- There is a lot of controlled breathing with this exercise – take care you do not over breathe.
- Do not allow the buttock muscles to join in.
- Keep your jaw relaxed.
- Don't take your shoulders up to the top floor too – keep them down and relaxed.
- Try not to grip around your hips.
- Keep the pelvis and spine quite still.

The Emergency Stop

Aim

Stress incontinence is surprisingly common. The following exercise will help you to cope with emergencies such as coughing or sneezing.

Action

1. Simply lift the whole of the pelvic floor, tightening it all quickly as if in an emergency. Hold for about 5 seconds, then release – keep breathing.
2. Repeat 6 times.

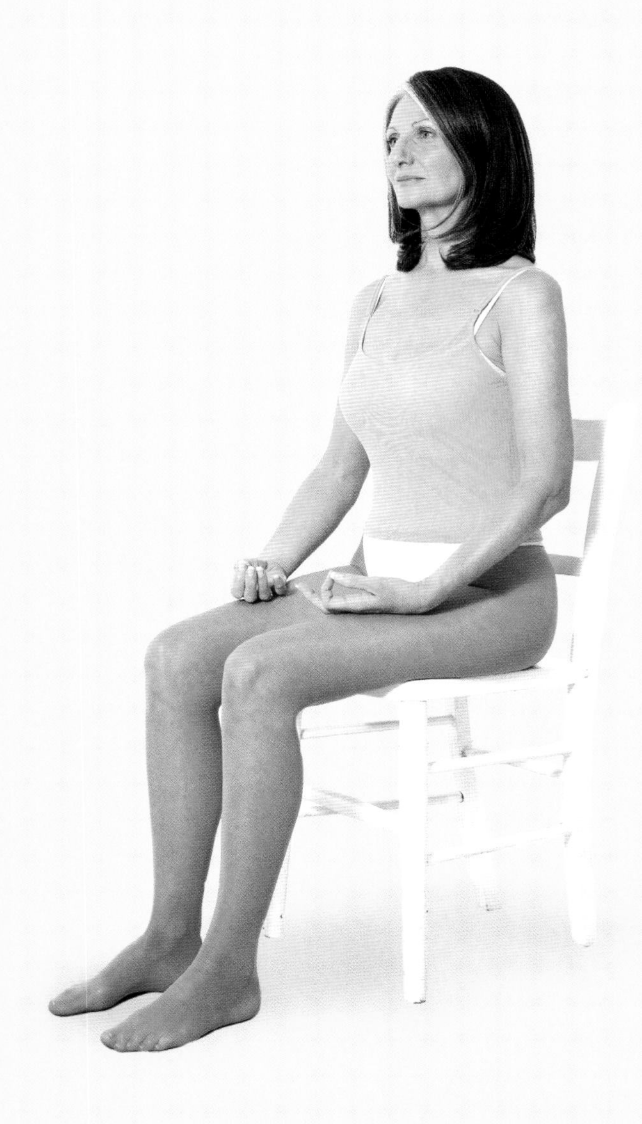

Hip Flexor Stretch

Aim
To lengthen the hip flexors gently.

If you sit all day, it is likely that your hip flexor muscles will shorten. If they do, this will affect the angle of your pelvis pulling it forward, which can put strain on the low back.

Starting Position
Lie in the Relaxation Position (page 26).

IMPORTANT NOTE

You will need to change position regularly every 3 minutes if you are in your last two trimesters.

Action

1. Breathe in wide and full to prepare.
2. Breathe out and zip up and hollow. Keeping that sense of hollowness in the pelvis, hinge the right knee up to your chest, dropping the thigh bone down into the hip joint.
3. Breathe in, as you clasp the right leg under the thigh so that the joint is not compressed.
4. Breathe out, still zipping and hollowing, and stretch the left leg along the floor. Your lower back should remain in neutral. If it arches, bend the left knee back up again a little. Hold this stretch for 5 breaths.
5. Breathe in as you slide the left leg back.
6. Breathe out and zip up and hollow, as you lower the right foot to the floor, keeping the abdominals engaged.
7. Repeat twice on each side, keeping your shoulders relaxed and down.

Watchpoints

- Check the position of the upper body, elbows open, breastbone soft, shoulder blades down into the back, neck released.
- Are you in neutral?

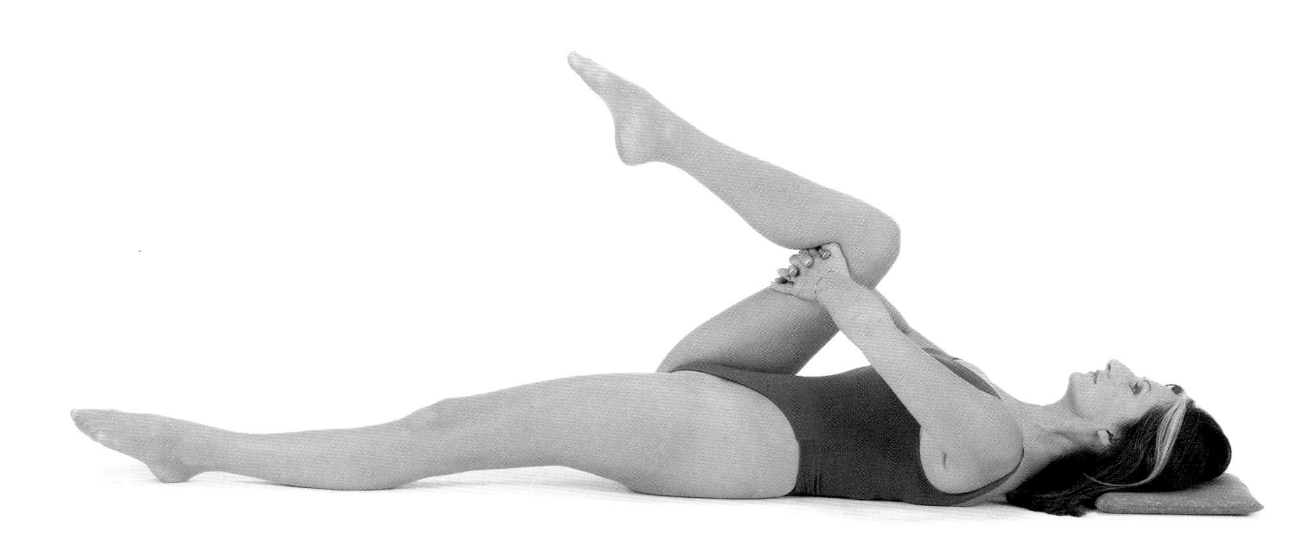

Double Knee Fold: Level One

This exercise looks deceptively easy, but is in fact one of the hardest in the book! Bringing the knees towards the chest one at a time, without allowing the lower abdominals to bulge and without losing neutral, requires excellent core stability. This exercise is a part of the preparation for many classical exercises such as the Single Leg Stretch (page 75) or the Hundred (page 78).

We have given you two levels of difficulty. It is easier to learn Double Knee Folds in reverse – that is, lowering the feet to the floor rather than lifting them off. It gives you some idea of the strength and control you need to do Level Two.

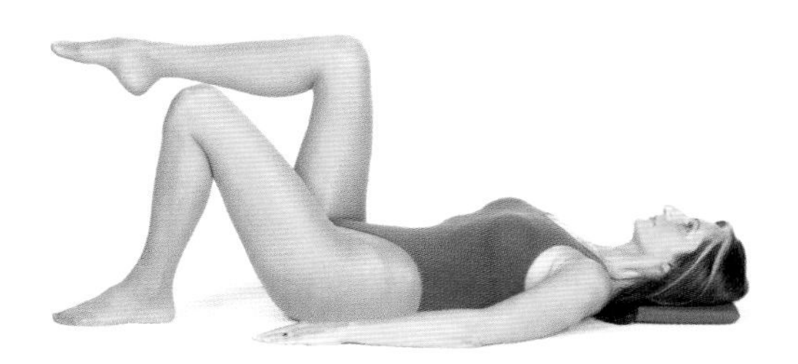

Starting Position

Lie in the Relaxation Position (page 26).

Action

1. Breathe in wide and full to prepare.
2. Breathe out, zip up and hollow and stay zipped and hollowed throughout. Fold one knee up, staying in neutral and keeping the lower abdominals hollow as for Knee Folds (page 55).
3. Breathe in and lightly take hold of the raised knee, with one or both hands.
4. Breathe out and fold the second knee up so that both knees are now bent at an angle so that it looks as though you are sitting on a chair (lying on your back, of course). Line your feet up so that the toes are lightly touching but the knees stay hip-width apart.
5. Now for the hard bit! Let go of the knee. Breathe in and lengthen through the spine and check that your pelvis is in neutral and that your low back feels anchored (use your zip).
6. Breathe out, still zipped, and slowly lower one foot to the floor – do not allow the abdominals to bulge or lose neutral.
7. Breathe in, then out, and slowly lower the other foot.
8. Repeat 6 times, alternating which leg you raise and lower first.

Watchpoints

- You will be surprised at how the body tries to cheat and use everything other than the lower abdominals to stabilize you – be aware of this and keep your neck and shoulders relaxed.

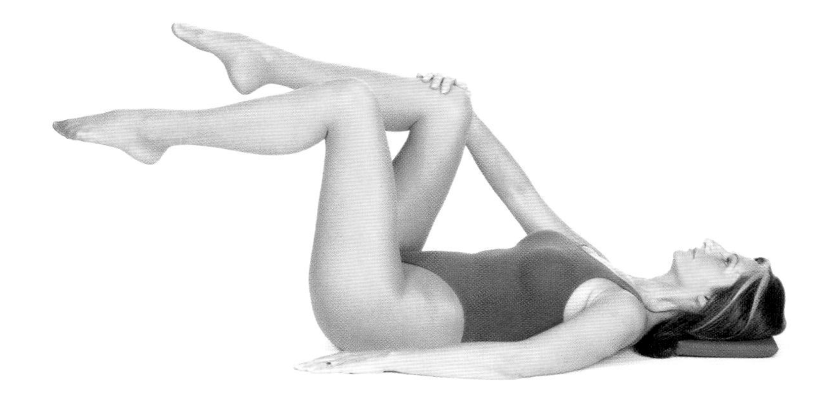

Double Knee Fold: Level Two

This is a challenging exercise.

Starting Position
Lie in the Relaxation Position (page 26).

Action
1. Breathe in wide and full to prepare.
2. Breathe out, zip up and hollow and stay zipped and hollowed throughout. Fold one knee up. The lower abdominals stay hollow. The pelvis is in neutral.
3. Breathe in wide and full.
4. Breathe out and fold the other knee up. Stay neutral.
5. Breathe in wide.
6. Breathe out and lower the first leg you raised.
7. Breathe in, then out, and lower the second leg.
8. Repeat 6 times, alternating which leg you raise and lower first.

Watchpoints
- Keep your sacrum square on the mat, the tailbone down.
- Keep the back of your neck long.
- Your lower abdominals must stay hollow and scooped throughout.
- Your back must stay firmly anchored to the mat.

IMPORTANT NOTE

You will need to change position regularly every 3 minutes if you are in your last two trimesters.

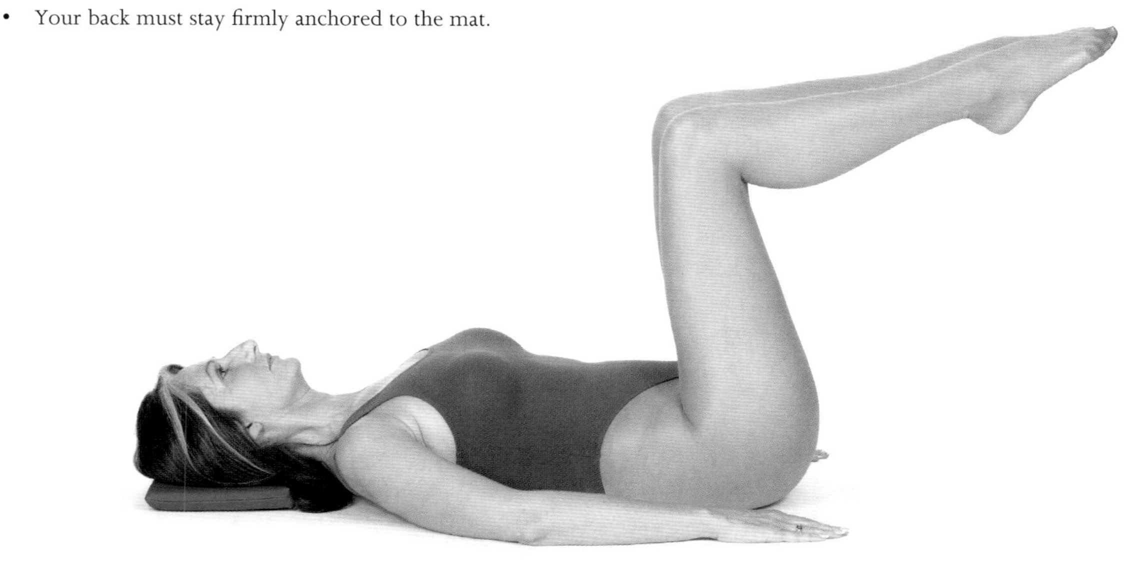

Single Leg Stretch: Level One

There are two levels to this fantastic classical exercise.

Aim

To strengthen the abdominals and challenge core stability and co-ordination skills.

Starting Position

Lie in the Relaxation Position (page 26).

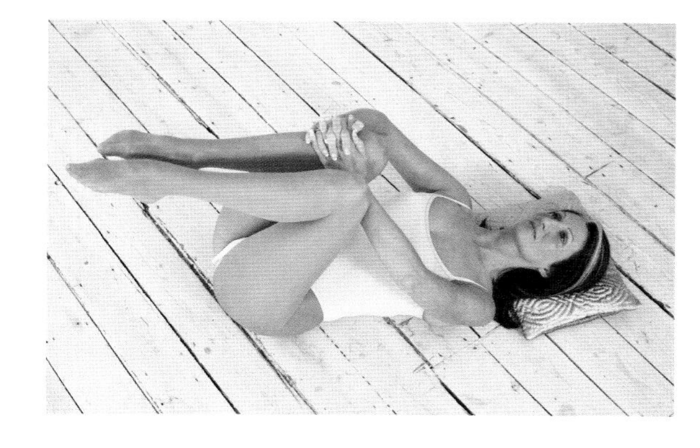

Action

1. Breathe in wide and full to prepare.
2. Breathe out, zip up and hollow, and Double Knee Fold (page 74) one leg at a time.
3. Breathe in and lightly clasp your right leg below the knee with both hands. Keep your elbows open and your breastbone soft. Your shoulder blades stay down into your back. Your neck is released.
4. Breathe out, zip up and hollow, and slowly straighten the left leg straight up into the air. Keep your back anchored into the floor.
5. Breathe in and bend the leg back in.
6. Hold the left leg now and straighten the right leg up into the air.
7. Repeat 8 times with each leg.
8. Do not allow the leg to fall away from you; your back must stay anchored to the floor. When this becomes easy – and only when – you may try the more advanced version.

Watchpoints

- Do not allow the back to arch.
- Keep your neck released.
- Your leg must go straight up and not drop, or you will strain your abdominals.

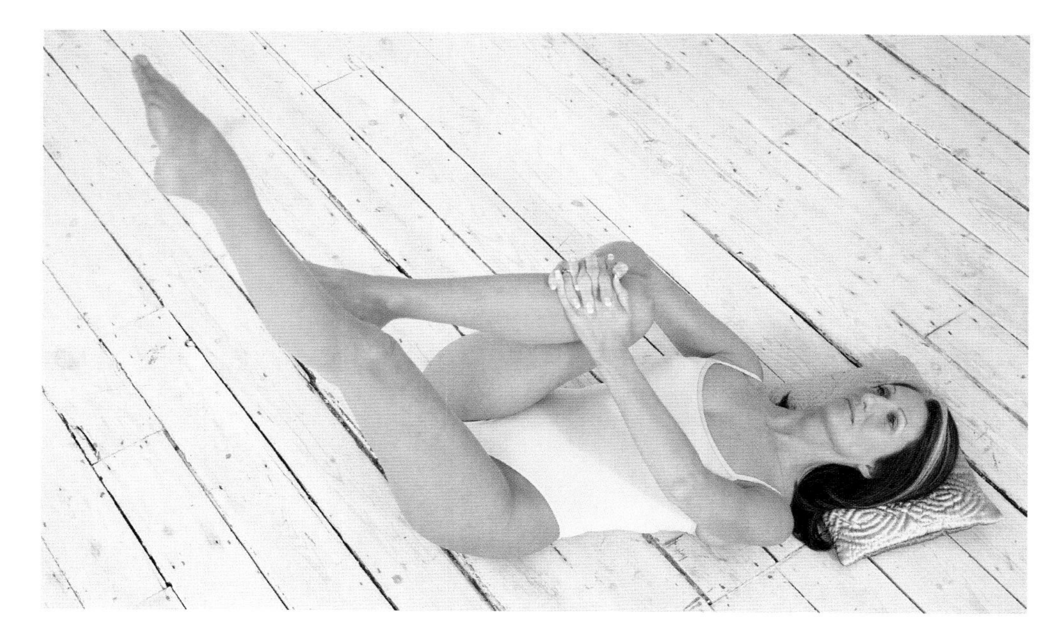

Single Leg Stretch: Level Two

This has to be the best abdominal exercise there is! You might like to familiarize yourself with the hand position before you start the exercise because it is a challenge to your co-ordination skills. The role the hands play is to bring the knee towards the chest while still keeping the upper body open.

- Sit tall on your mat with your knees bent and slightly apart in front of you.
- Put your right hand on the outside of your right knee or your calf (this will depend on your arm length when you do the full exercise).
- Place your left hand on the inside of your right knee.
- Your elbows are open, your breastbone is soft and your shoulder blades down into your back – your arms form a soft open 'C' shape.
- Now, change sides and place your left hand on the outside of your left knee or calf and your right hand on the inside of your left knee.

Practise this a few times to lock it into your memory banks before trying the complete movement.

IMPORTANT NOTE

This version is not suitable for during pregnancy.

Starting Position
Lie in the Relaxation Position (page 26).

Action

1. Breathe in to prepare.
2. Breathe out, zip up and hollow and stay zipped and hollowed throughout. Double Knee Fold (page 74). The toes should just touch; the knees are hip-width apart and parallel. Keep your feet softly pointed. Place your hands on the outsides of your knees or the outsides of your calves.
3. Breathe in and check that your elbows are open to enable the chest to expand fully. Your shoulder blades are down into your back.
4. Breathe out and soften your breastbone. Curl the upper body off the floor. The chin is tucked in.
5. Breathe in and move the left hand to the inside of the right knee.
6. Breathe out and slowly stretch your left leg away in parallel, so that it is at an angle of 45° to the floor. The toes are softly pointed.
7. Breathe in wide and full, as you begin to bend the leg back to your chest, bringing it back in line with your shoulder.
8. Change hands so that your left hand is on the outside of your left leg, your right hand is on the inside of your left knee.
9. Breathe out and stretch the right leg away in parallel. Do not take it too close to the floor.
10. Breathe in as the leg returns.
11. Repeat 10 stretches on each leg, making sure that you have a strong centre throughout and that your shoulder blades stay down into your back, your elbows open.

Watchpoints

- Keep zipping and hollowing throughout, and do not allow the back to arch. The pelvis stays neutral.
- Keep your neck released and the upper body open. The shoulder blades stay down.
- Make sure you keep the length on both sides of your waist, do not allow one side to shorten.
- When you extend the leg, lengthen it away from the hip joint – a long, long leg.

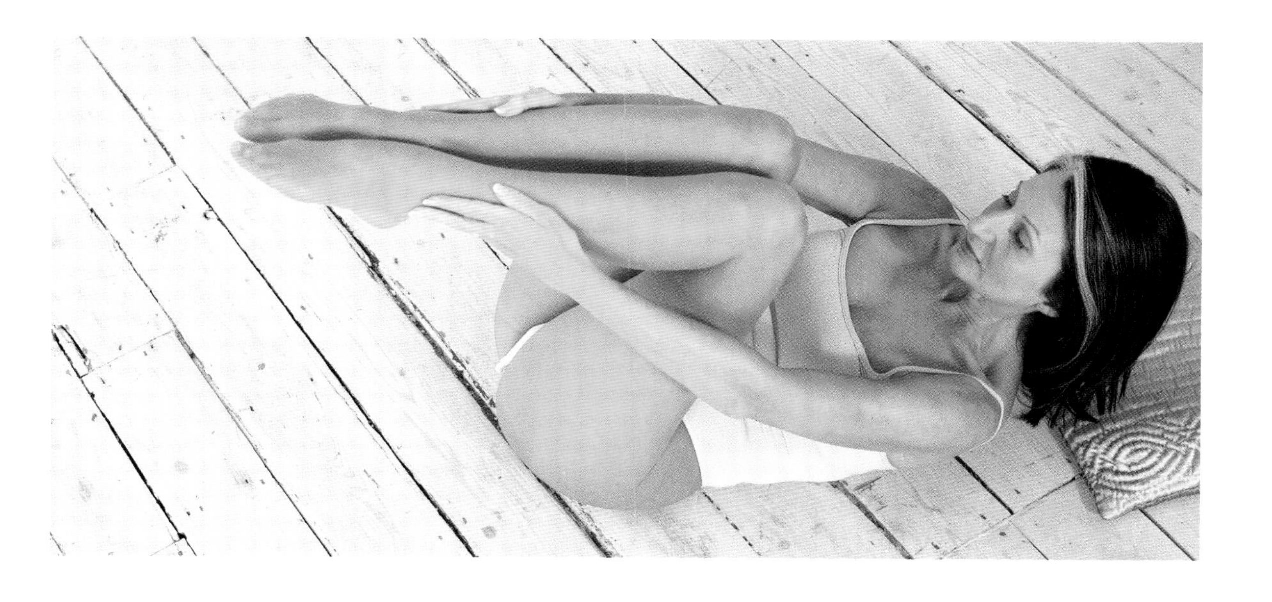

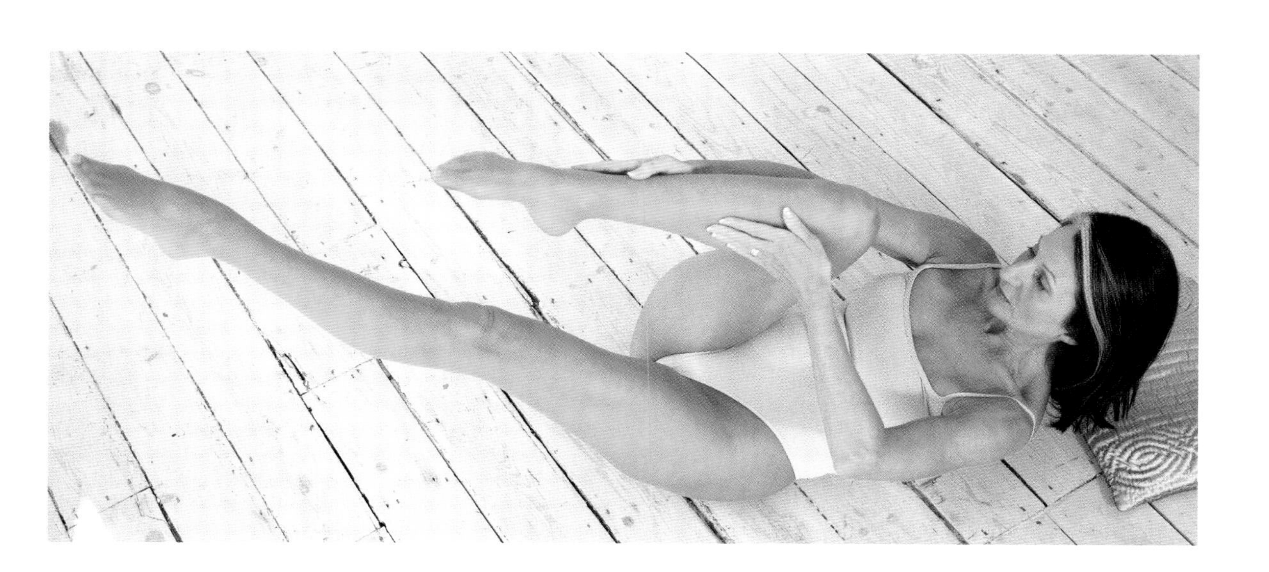

The Hundred (Stages One to Three)

Stage One is beginners; Stage Two is intermediate; Stage Three is advanced.

Aim

To learn the breathing pattern of the Hundred, which involves lateral lower ribcage breathing to a set rhythm. To strengthen the pectoral muscles. To master stabilizing the shoulder blades. To strengthen the abdominals.

The Hundred is one of the classical Pilates exercises. It used to be the warm-up exercise for mat classes. Well, it certainly warms you up! We have broken the exercise down into manageable bite-sized chunks. When you have mastered one stage, you may proceed to the next. This first stage tackles the breathing pattern, which stimulates the circulatory system, oxygenating the blood.

Please take advice if you have neck, respiratory or heart problems.

Stage One: Breathing Preparation

1. Lie in the Relaxation Position (page 26) zip and hollow. Place your hands on your lower ribcage. Breathe in wide and full into your sides and back for a count of 5. Breathe out and zip up and hollow, for a count of 5.
2. Repeat 5 times, trying to stay zipped and hollowed for both the in- and out-breaths. If you find the count of 5 too difficult try a count of 3.
3. Extend your arms alongside your body, palms down, wrists straight and reaching away through your fingers. Breath in, then out and pump your arms up and down no more than 15 cm (6 inches) off the floor for a count of 5 full in-breaths and 5 full out-breaths, keep your shoulders down and your fingers lengthening away. The movement is as if you are splashing water.
4. Repeat 5 times.

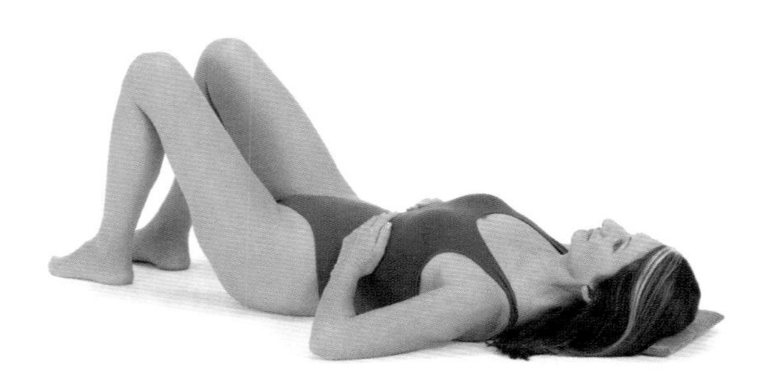

Stage One, Actions 1 and 2

IMPORTANT NOTE

You will need to change position regularly every 3 minutes if you are in your last two trimesters.

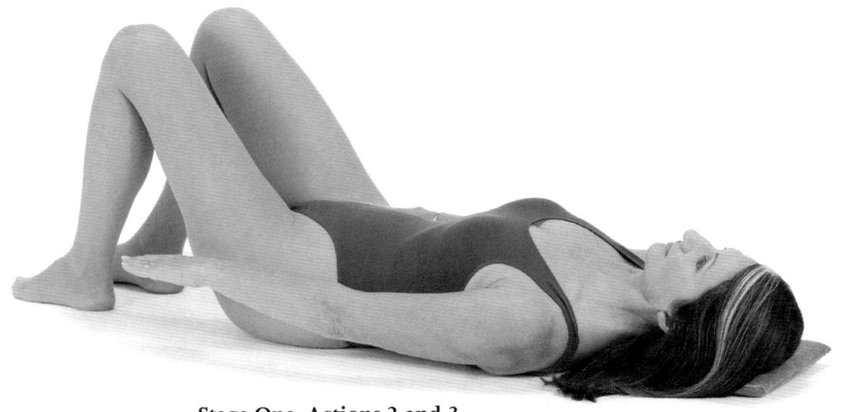

Stage One, Actions 2 and 3

Stage Two: Starting Position

Lie in the Relaxation Position (page 26). Double Knee Fold (page 74), toes lightly touching but knees hip-width apart. Your arms are extended alongside your body, palms down, wrists straight.

Action

1. Breathe in wide and full.
2. Breathe out, zip up and hollow and stay zipped and hollowed throughout. Curl up remembering the directions from Curl Ups (page 68).
3. Breathing in and out wide into your sides and back, pump your arms up and down, no more than 15 centimetres (6 inches) off the floor for a count of 5 for the in-breath and 5 for the out-breath. The shoulder blades stay down, with the fingers lengthening away.
4. Repeat up to 10 times, then slowly lower your head and, still zipping and hollowing, Double Knee Fold down, one leg at a time.

Watchpoints

- Your breathing should be comfortable. Do not over breathe. If you feel light-headed, take a break.
- As you beat the arms be aware of any unnecessary tension in your neck, keep the neck released.
- Your shoulder blades should stay down into your back as your arms lengthen away.
- Keep a sense of openness in the upper body. It is very easy to close the shoulders in, rounding them. Keep them opened out. The breastbone is soft and the neck released.

IMPORTANT NOTE

This is not suitable for trimesters 2 or 3.

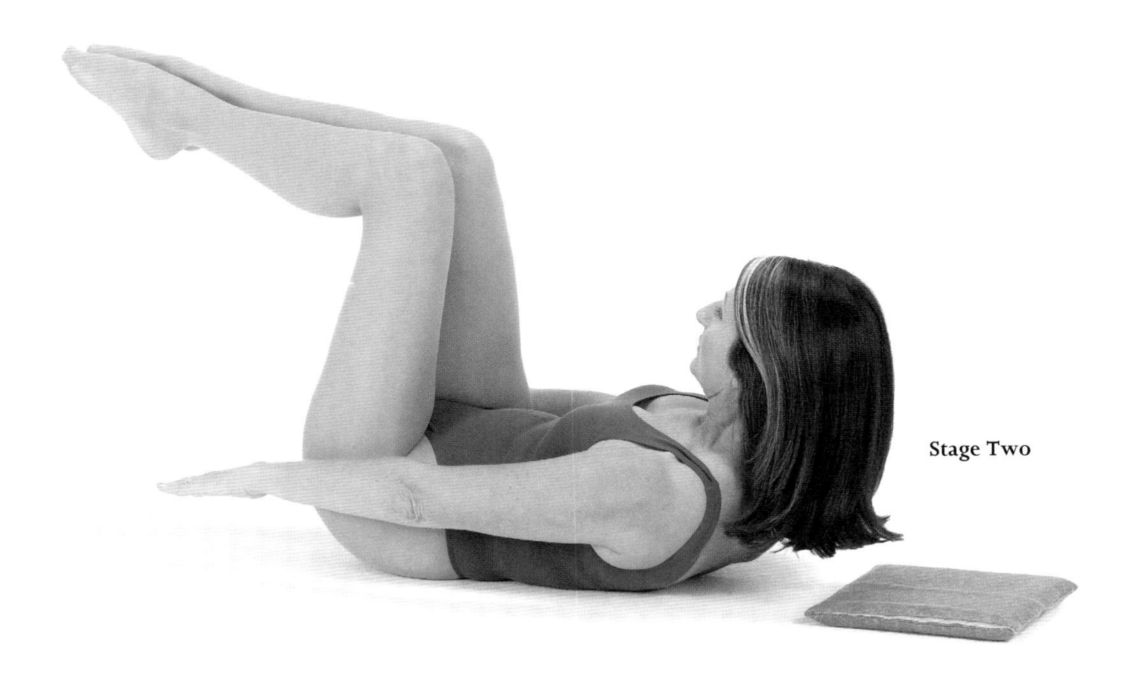

Stage Two

Stage Three: Starting Position

As for Stage Two.

Action

1. Breathe in wide and full to prepare.
2. Breathe out, zip up and hollow and stay zipped and hollowed throughout. Curl the upper body up off the floor, remembering everything you learnt for Curl Ups (page 68): chin gently tucked forward, jaw relaxed, breastbone soft, neck released.
3. Breathe in and then out, as you straighten the legs into the air as high as is comfortable. You may still keep them bent if you find this difficult. Do not allow them to fall away from you, because this may cause your back to arch. Your back must stay anchored to the mat. Have your feet softly pointed.
4. Start the breathing and pumping action of the arms, which you mastered in the last stage. Breathe in wide for 5 beats and out for 5 beats. Keep the shoulder blades down and the fingertips lengthening away.
5. Repeat up to 10 times until you reach 100, then slowly bend your knees to your chest and lower your head. Double Knee Fold (page 74) down.

Watchpoints

- Return to the floor if you feel any strain in your neck.
- To prevent strain and engage the deep stabilizers, keep your chin gently tucked in but not squashed. Your line of focus should be between your thighs. The back of your neck remains long, the front relaxed.
- You must keep breathing wide into your lower ribcage or you will become breathless. If you do feel breathless, stop at once.
- Keep a sense of width in your upper body. Do not close the shoulders in; keep the upper body open, the breastbone soft.

IMPORTANT NOTE

This version is not suitable for use in pregnancy.

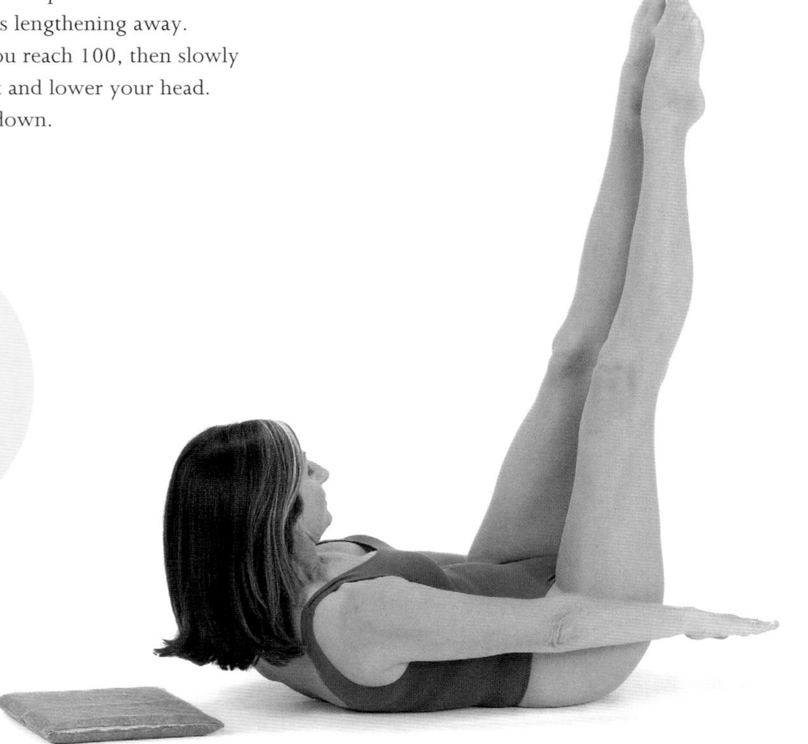

Stage Three

Hip Rolls

Aim

To work the obliques, which define your waist. To teach you how to rotate the spine safely with stability and length. The tennis ball ensures that you keep good alignment of the knees and hips.

Equipment

A tennis ball.

Level One (Beginners): Starting Position

Lie in the Relaxation Position (page 26) and bring your feet together, lining up the bones. Put the tennis ball between your knees. Place your arms, palms up, out to the sides just below shoulder height.

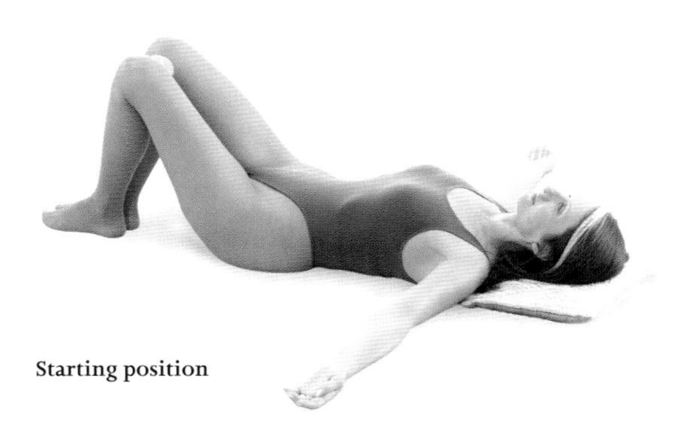

Starting position

Action

1. Breathe in wide and full to prepare.
2. Breathe out, zip up and hollow and stay zipped and hollowed throughout. Roll your head to the left, your knees to the right. Only roll a little way to start with – you can go further each time if it is comfortable. Keep your left shoulder down on the floor, and turn the palm of your left hand down. Your feet stay on the floor.
3. Breathe in then breathe out; use your strong centre to bring the knees back to the Starting Position. The head moves back as well. The palm turns up.
4. Repeat 8 times in each direction. Think of rolling each part of your back off the floor in sequence and then returning the back of the ribcage, the waist, the small of your back and the buttock to the floor.

Watchpoints

- Your feet will make an action a bit like a plane banking. Keep the inner borders of the feet glued together.
- Keep working those abdominals. Do not simply allow the weight of the legs to pull you over.

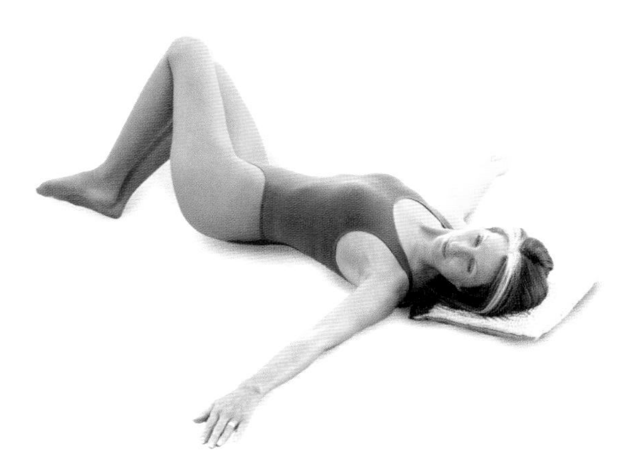

NOTE

Please take advice if you have a disc-related injury.

Level Two (Intermediate): Starting Position

Lie in the Relaxation Position (page 26). Double Knee Fold (page 74). Place the tennis ball between your knees. Take your arms out to your sides, just below shoulder height, palms up this time. Your feet are softly pointed.

Action

1. Breathe in wide and full to prepare, then, as you breathe out, zip up and hollow and stay zipped and hollowed thoughout. Slowly lower your legs towards the floor on your right side, turning your head to the left and your left palm down. Keep the left shoulder down on the ground. Keep the knees in line.
2. Breathe in and breathe out. Use your girdle of strength to bring your legs back to the middle. The head returns to the centre, the palm turns up again.
3. Breathe in and then out, and repeat the twisting movement to the opposite side.
4. Repeat 10 times to each side.

Watchpoints

- Keep the opposite shoulder firmly down on the floor.
- Keep the knees in line. Don't go too far unless you can control it.
- Use the abdominals at all times – feel as though you are moving the legs from the stomach.
- It is a sideways lateral movement, don't deviate.
- Do not force the neck the opposite way; allow it to roll comfortably. Keep it long.

IMPORTANT NOTE

Do not attempt this version if you are already pregnant.

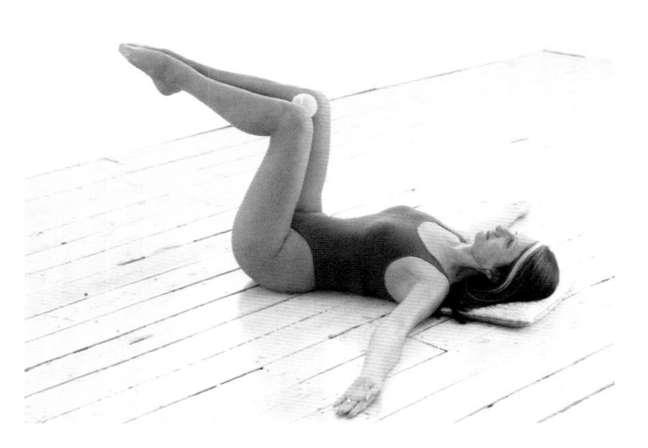

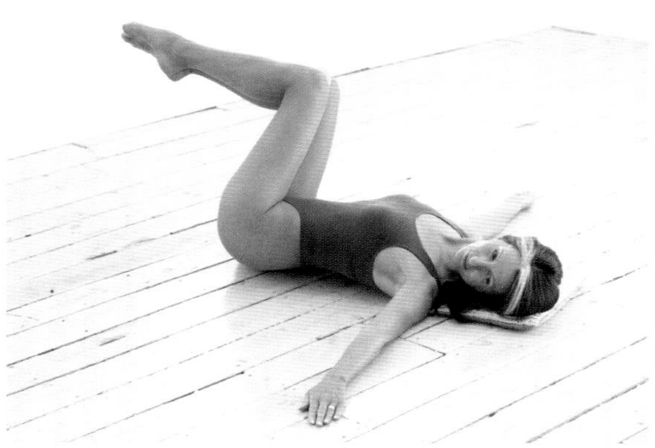

Roll Downs

This is always a favourite because it helps to release tension in the body. It is fine to do this in pregnancy – you are only limited by the size of your bump. We have given two versions: using a wall and free-standing.

Aim
To release tension in the spine, the shoulders and the upper body. To mobilize the spine, creating flexibility and strength, and achieving segmental control. To teach correct use of stabilizing abdominals when bending.

As you roll back up think of rebuilding the spinal column, stacking each vertebra on top of each other to lengthen out the spine.

NOTE

Take advice before attempting this exercise if you have a back problem, especially if it is disc-related. If you feel dizzy stop immediately. Avoid Roll Downs if you have low blood pressure or feel nauseous.

Rolling Down a Wall

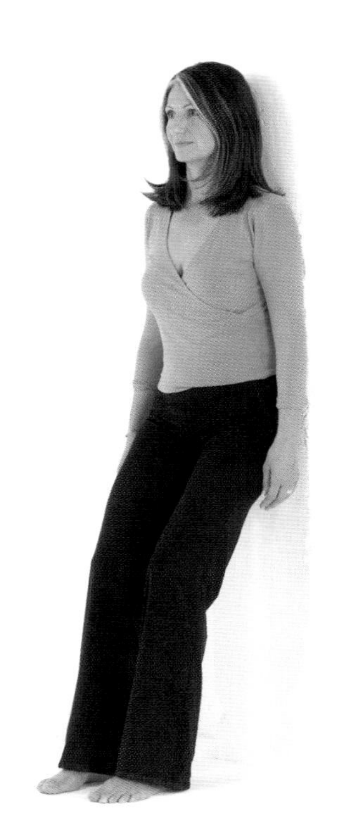

Starting Position

Stand about 45 centimetres (18 inches) away from a wall (the distance really depends on your height, but you should feel comfortable). Bend your knees so that from the side you look as if you are sitting on a bar stool! Have your feet hip-width apart and in parallel, your weight evenly balanced on both feet. Be sure that you cannot slip. Check that you are not rolling your feet in or out. Take an extra breath any time you need to.

Action

1. Breathe in to prepare and lengthen up through the spine. Release the head and neck.
2. Breathe out, zip up and hollow, and drop your chin to your chest and allow the weight of your head to make you roll slowly forward, head released, arms hanging, centre strong, knees soft. If you have a back problem, you may like to begin by sliding your hands down your thighs.
3. Breathe in as you hang, really letting your head and arms release.
4. Breathe out, keeping firmly zipped up and hollowed, as you drop your tailbone down, directing your pubic bone forward and rotating your pelvis backwards as you slowly come up the wall, rolling through the spine bone by bone.
5. Repeat 6 times.

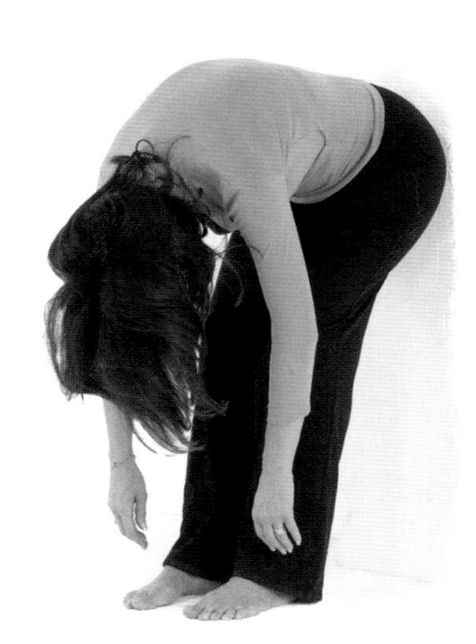

Watchpoints

- You may like to take an extra breath during the exercise. This is fine, but please try to breathe out as you move the spine.
- Make sure you go down centrally and do not sway over to one side. When you are down, check where your hands are in relation to your feet.
- Do not roll the feet in or out. Keep the weight evenly balanced and try not to lean forward on to the front of your feet or back on to the heels.

Free-Standing Roll Downs

Starting Position

Stand with your feet hip-width apart and parallel and your weight evenly balanced on both feet. Check that you are not rolling your feet in or out. Soften your knees. Find your neutral pelvis position, but keep the tailbone lengthening down. Take an extra breath any time you need to.

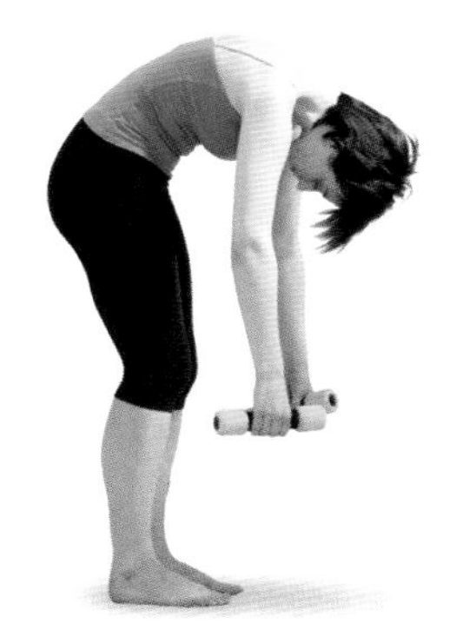

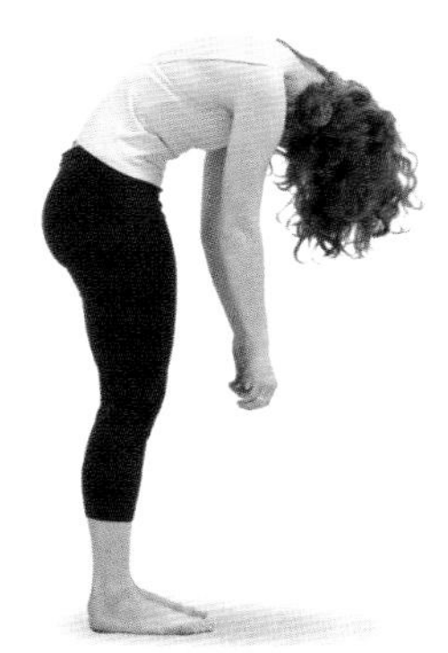

Action

1. Breathe in to prepare and lengthen up through the spine; release the head and neck.
2. Breathe out and zip up and hollow. Drop your chin to your chest and allow the weight of your head to make you slowly roll forward, head released, arms hanging, centre strong, knees soft.
3. Breathe in as you hang, really letting your head and arms hang. Try not to lean forward or back; stay central.
4. Breathe out, staying firmly zipped, as you drop your tailbone down, directing your pubic bone forward and rotating your pelvis backwards as you slowly come up to standing tall, rolling through the spine bone by bone.
5. Repeat 6 times.

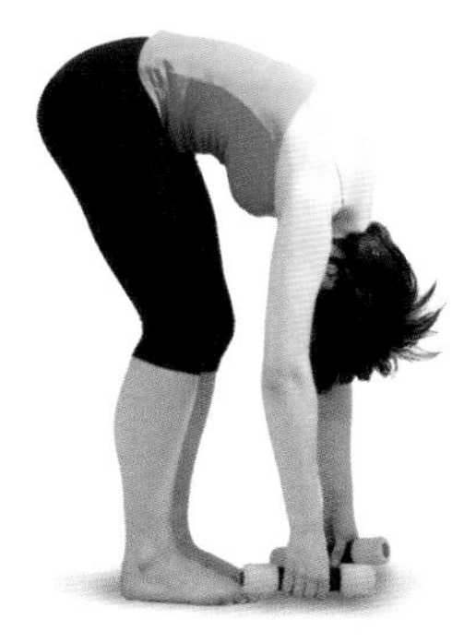

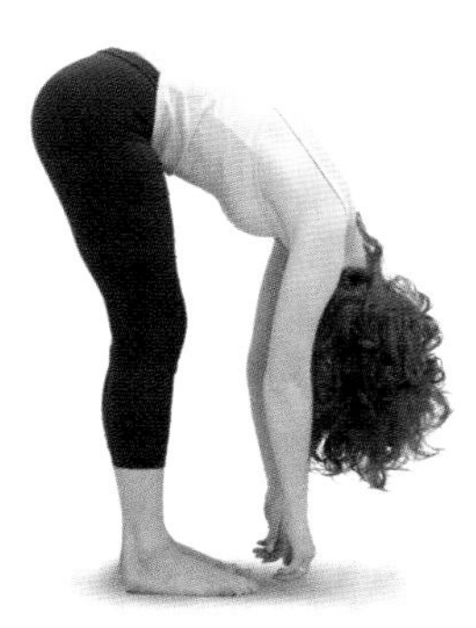

Watchpoints

- You may like to take an extra breath during the exercise. This is fine, but please try to breathe out as you move the spine.
- Make sure you go down centrally and do not sway over to one side. When you are down, check where your hands are in relation to your feet.
- Do not roll the feet in or out. Keep the weight evenly balanced and try not to lean forward on to the front of your feet or back on to the heels.

Variation

Try holding light weights of 0.5 kilos (1 pound) each weight as you do this; it helps relax the shoulders.

Sitting Side Reach

A gentle side stretch which feels really good.

We all have a preferred way of sitting cross-legged. It helps to balance the body if you sometimes cross your legs the other way.

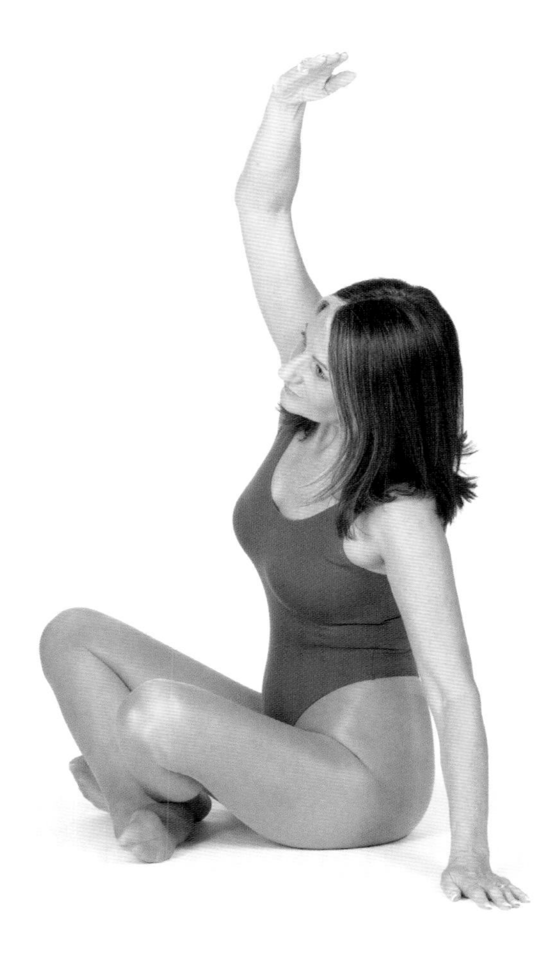

Equipment
A rolled-up towel (optional).

Starting Position
Sit with a rolled-up towel under your bottom if this is more comfortable. Sit tall with your legs crossed. Make sure you are sitting on your sitting bones and that the natural curves of the spine are maintained. Rest your arms on the floor beside you.

Action

1. Breathe in wide to prepare and lengthen up through the spine.
2. Breath out, zip up and hollow, and stay zipped throughout. Float one arm up, remembering what you learnt in Floating Arms (page 59).
3. Breathe in, then out, and reach up and across, lifting up out of the waist rather than simply reaching through the shoulders. Keep both buttocks firmly on the mat.
4. Breathe in and return to centre.
5. Breathe out and float the arm back down.
6. Repeat twice to each side, then change the way you are sitting cross-legged and repeated twice more to each side.

Watchpoints

- Try not to lean forward or back, but go directly to the side.
- Keep your head in a line with your spine.

Abductor Lifts

When you have completed all the leg exercises – Abductor and Adductor Lifts and Torpedo – on one side, turn over and repeat them on the other side.

Aim

This exercise is designed to strengthen the abductors (outer thigh) and the gluteals (buttocks). It also tones the upper leg and helps control cellulite.

This and the following exercise challenge your pelvic and lumbar stability, so you must be stable before you attempt them. Good preparation exercises are the Pelvic Stability exercises (page 54).

Equipment

Practise this and the following exercise firstly without weights until you are totally familiar with them and they cause you no discomfort. You may then strap leg weights of up to 1.5 kilos (about 3 pounds) on to your ankles. Start with the lightest weight. A flat cushion.

IMPORTANT NOTE

While you are pregnant or post-natal, do not use weights.

NOTE

If you are lucky enough to lack natural padding around your hip, you may find it uncomfortable to lie like this. If so, just put a small piece of foam, or a flat, firm cushion underneath your hip.

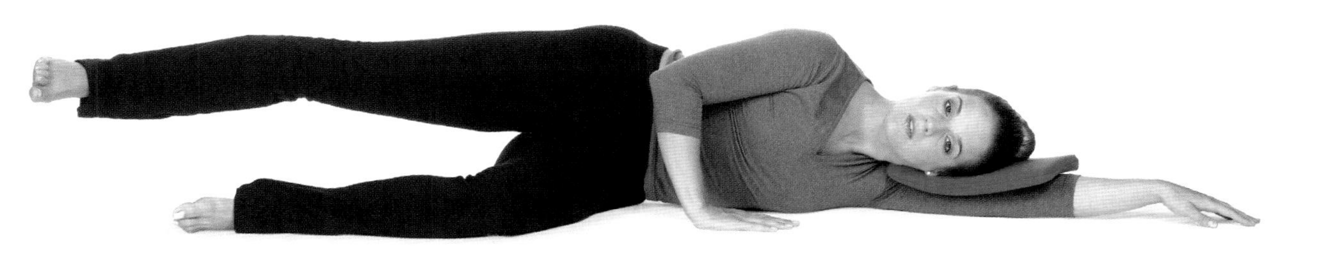

Starting Position

Lie on your left side in a straight line – this is crucial, so, if you like, you can lie up against a wall to check your alignment. Don't lean on the wall! Remember, neutral, please. Your left arm is stretched out and your head rests on it. You may place a cushion between your ear and your arm so that the head is at a right angle to the spine. Bend both legs in front of you at an angle of just under 90°. Use your right arm to support yourself in front. Throughout the exercise, keep lifting the waist off the floor and maintain the length in the trunk. If you are already pregnant you may like to support your bump with a cushion.

Action

1. Zip up and hollow and stay zipped and hollowed throughout. Straighten your top leg so that it is in a line with your hip and about 12 centimetres (5 inches) off the floor. Be careful not to take it behind you! Rotate the leg in very slightly from the hip; the pelvis stays still. Flex the foot towards your face.
2. Breathe out as you slowly lift the leg about 15 centimetres (6 inches), then breathe in and lower.
3. Raise and lower the leg 10 times, without returning it to the floor. You are breathing out as you raise it and in as you lower it.
4. Bend the leg to rest on the bent one underneath.

Watchpoints

- Keep zipping and hollowing so you protect the low back and prevent it from arching or the waist from dropping down to the floor.
- Lengthen the heel as far away as possible from the hip . . . long, long leg.
- Keep the rotation inward from the hip. Be careful not to turn it in just from the ankle. It is a small rotation.
- Keep lifting the waist off the floor and lengthening in the body . . . long, long waist.
- Your pelvis should remain absolutely still; do not allow it to roll forward or rock around.
- Don't forget to keep the upper body open and the shoulder blades down into your back. Do not allow yourself to roll forward.

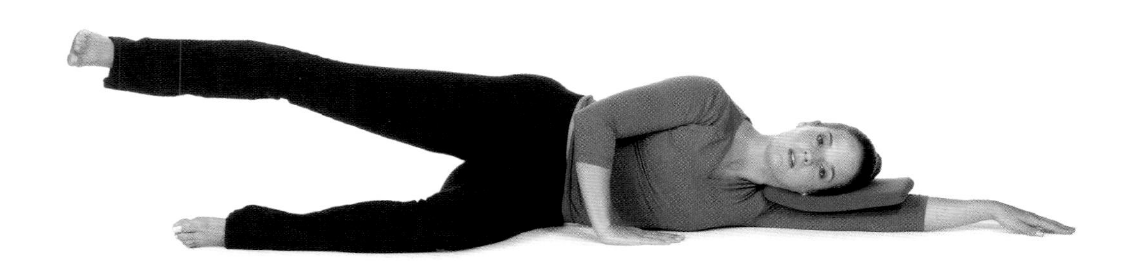

Adductor Lifts

Aim
To tone the inner thigh muscles. To learn pelvic stability.

Equipment
As for Abductor Lifts (page 87), plus a large cushion.

Starting Position
Lie on your left side as for Abductor Lifts and if you are already pregnant support your bump with a cushion. Straighten the bottom leg away a little in front of you, turning it out from the hip joint. Point or flex the foot; either is fine. Bend your top knee and rest it on top of a large pillow. The idea is for your pelvis to stay square and not drop forward.

IMPORTANT NOTE

While you are pregnant or post-natal, do not use weights

Action
1. Breathe in wide and full to prepare.
2. Keeping the leg turned out from the hip, long and straight, breathe out. Zip up and hollow and stay zipped and hollowed throughout, as you slowly raise the underneath leg as high as you can without losing neutral. Keep lengthening it away. Do not allow your waist to sink into the floor; keep working it.
3. Breathe in as you lower the leg.
4. Repeat up to 20 times.

Watchpoints
- Keep zipping and hollowing throughout.
- Don't let the waist sag; keep lengthening it.
- Check that you are moving the whole leg together and not just twisting from the knee.
- Don't let your foot sickle (curl) round to help you come up further. The action must be from the inside of the thigh.
- Check that your upper body stays open and your shoulder blades down. Do not roll forward.

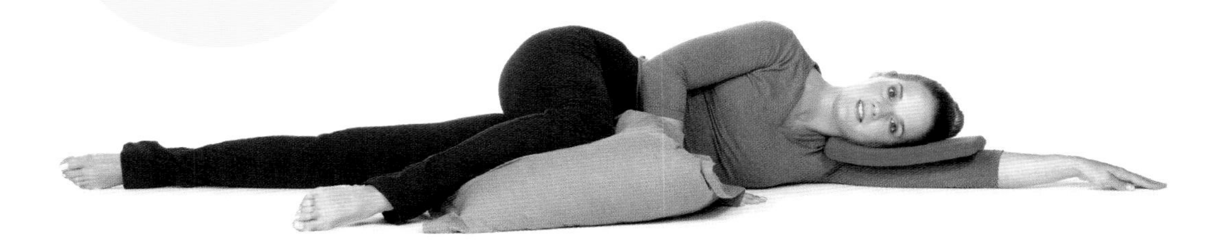

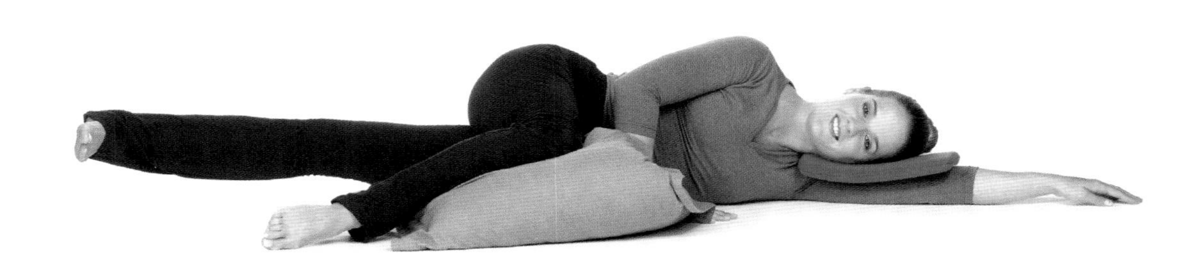

Torpedo

This is not suitable in your second and third trimesters.

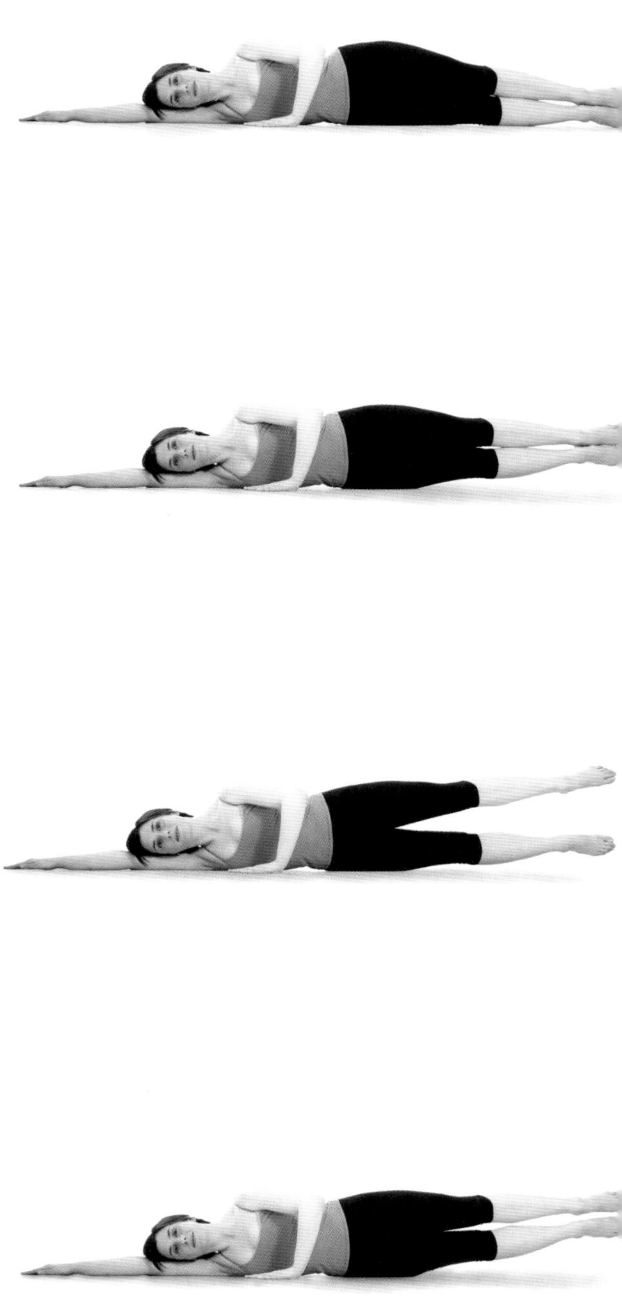

Aim
To test your core stability, balance and alignment.

Starting Position
Lie in a straight line on your right side – shoulder over shoulder, hip over hip, ankle over ankle. Rest your head on your extended, underneath arm. Put your other arm on the floor in front of you to support you. Your hand will be in a line with your chest, your shoulder blades are down into the back, elbow open. Take care not to have your legs behind your bodyline.

Action

1. Breathe out and zip up and hollow.
2. Breathe in and keep zipping as you lift both legs together off the mat.
3. Breathe out and raise the upper leg a little higher while the underneath leg stays at the same height off the floor. Feel the length of the body from fingertips to toes, long and strong.
4. Breathe in and lower the top leg to touch the lower leg.
5. Breathe out and gently lower both legs back to the floor.
6. Repeat 5 times.

Watchpoints

- Try not to use the supporting arm to push yourself up.
- Make sure you maintain neutral pelvis and spine. Do not arch the back.
- Keep an open elbow on the supporting arm; the shoulder stays down.
- Really enjoy lengthening through the whole body, keeping a long waistline.

The Dart (Stage Two)

Aim

To strengthen the back muscles. To create awareness of the shoulder blades and to strengthen the muscles which stabilize them.

Equipment

A firm, flat cushion.

Starting Position

Lie on your front. You may put a flat cushion under your forehead to allow you to breathe. Your arms are down by your sides, your palms are facing your body. Your neck is long. Your legs are together, parallel, with your toes pointing.

IMPORTANT NOTE

This exercise is fine for when you are pregnant for as long as you can lie comfortably on your front.

Action

1. Breathe in to prepare and lengthen through the spine; tuck your chin in gently.
2. Breathe out, zip up and hollow and stay zipped and hollowed throughout. Slide your shoulder blades down into your back, lengthen your fingers away from you down towards your feet. The top of your head stays lengthening away from your tailbone. Keep looking straight down at the floor. Do not tip your head back. Squeeze your inner thighs together, but keep your feet on the floor. At the same time, slowly lift your upper body from the floor – don't come up too high, just a few centimetres. Use your mid-back muscles.
3. Breathe in and feel the length of the body from the tips of your toes to the top of your head.
4. Breathe out and lengthen, then lower back down.
5. Repeat 6 times.

Watchpoints

- Keep hollowing the lower abdominals.
- Do not strain the neck; it should feel released as your shoulders engage down into your back. Think of a swan's neck growing out between its wings.
- Remember to keep your feet on the floor.
- Stop if you feel at all uncomfortable in the low back. This exercise can also be done with the feet hip-width apart and the thigh and buttock muscles relaxed.

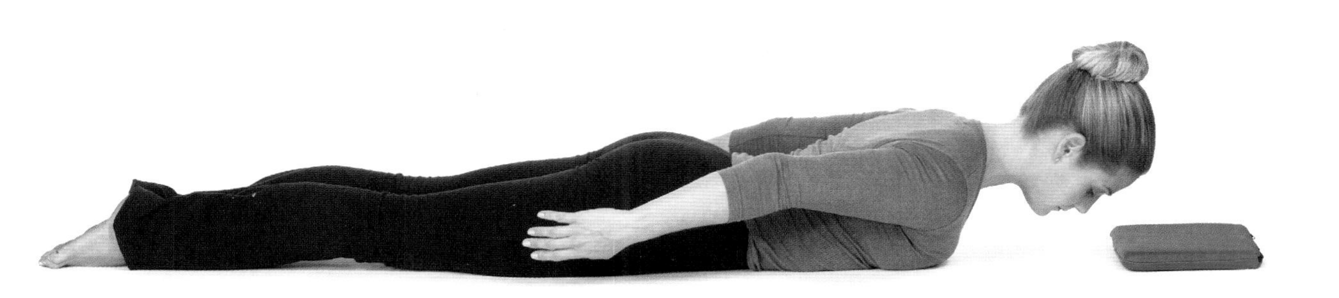

Front Leg Pull (*intermediate and advanced*)

This is a classical exercise that we have adapted. It requires good upper-body strength to perform it correctly.

Aim
To strengthen the upper body.

Starting Position
Come into four-point kneeling (page 50). Have your fingers pointing forward, your hands directly beneath your shoulders and your knees beneath your hips. Keep the natural curves of your back. Make sure that your body is long, the shoulders drawn down into your back and your head in a line with the body. You should feel as if your body is being pulled in two directions.

IMPORTANT NOTE

This exercise is not suitable for during pregnancy or if you have neck or shoulder problems.

Action (Intermediate)
1. Breathe in to prepare, zip up and hollow and stay zipped, hollowed and long throughout.
2. Breathe out. Slide one leg along the floor and tuck the toes under.
3. Breathe in, then out, and slide the other leg along the floor, tucking the toes under.
4. Bring your body into a plank position and hold for a breath. Press the heels away from you into the floor as far as you can, lengthening through your head.
5. On an out breath, return one leg at a time and return to the Starting Position.
6. Repeat once more.

Action (Advanced)
Follow directions 1–4 for intermediate.

1. Breathe in as you lift your right leg. The foot can be pointed or flexed but you must not move the hips or arch the back. Keep lengthening the head away and keep the ribcage flat. Press the left heel into the floor.
2. Breathe out as you lower the leg to the floor, still lengthening through the heel.
3. Repeat 5 times on each leg.

Watchpoints
- Keep your girdle of strength working; think of both scapular and pelvic stability.
- Keep the back of the neck long and released.
- Don't dip in the middle; use an image like an ironing board or a plank to help you.

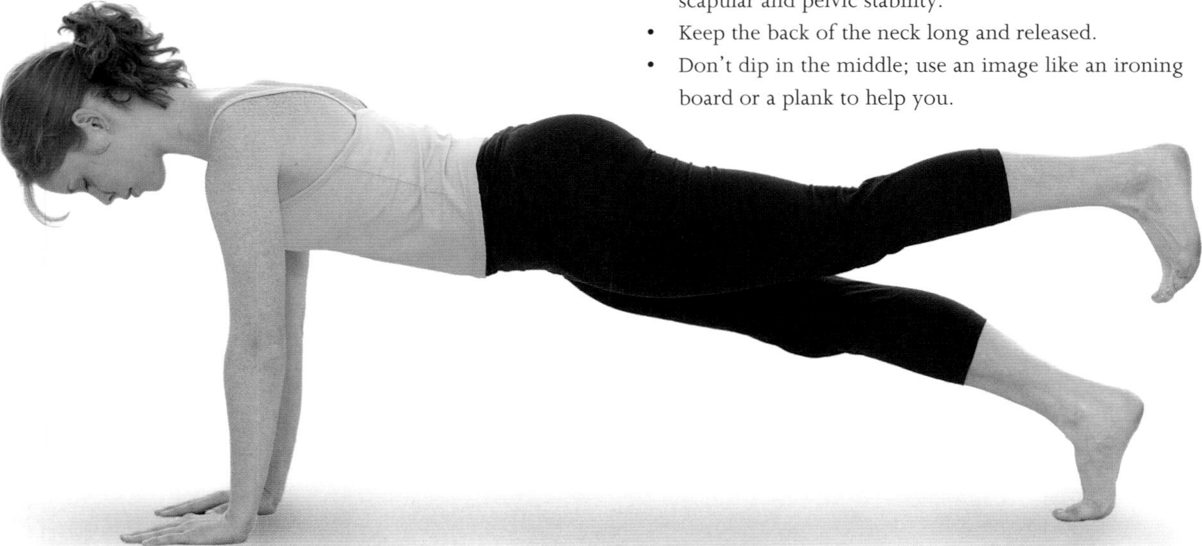

The Rest Position

Aim
This is a lovely way to stretch out the back, especially after doing back extensions or four-point kneeling exercises.

Equipment
While you are pregnant you will probably feel more comfortable if you rest on a few large pillows piled up in front of you. Try to keep your head higher than your bottom. A pillow under the knees will also help your leg circulation.

NOTE

Avoid the Rest Position if you have knee problems as you may compress the joint. It may help to put a pillow under the knees.

Action
1. Usually this exercise follows one in which you have been lying prone (on your front). So come up on to all fours and bring your feet together. Your knees stay apart. Slowly move back towards your buttocks. Do not raise your head or hands and come back to sit on your feet – not between them – with the back rounded. Rest and relax into this position. Leave the arms extended to give you a maximum stretch. Feel the expansion in the back of your ribcage as you breathe deeply into it.
2. The further apart the knees are, the more of a stretch you will feel in your inner thighs. With the knees further apart, you can really think of your chest sinking down into the floor.
3. Take 10 breaths in this position.

To Come Out of the Rest Position
As you breathe out, zip up and hollow and slowly unfurl. Think of dropping your tailbone down and bringing your pubic bone forward. Rebuild your spine vertebra by vertebra until you are upright.

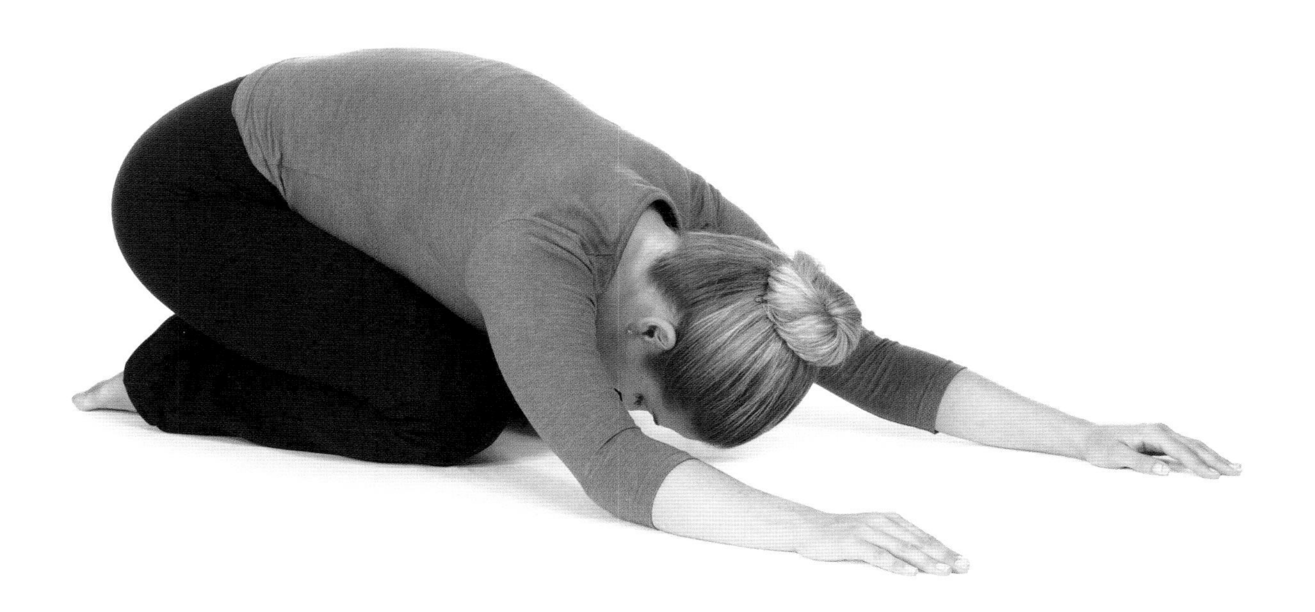

Workouts

There are 5 balanced workouts set out below. Each lasts approximately 20–30 minutes, and you should try to do all 5 workouts once each week.

The exercises are mainly drawn from this chapter but we have also added a few from earlier and later chapters which will make the workouts more varied. You can of course add any exercise from later in the book if you wish.

Work at whichever level you feel comfortable with, moving on to stage or level two of an exercise (where applicable) when you feel ready.

Workout One

The Full Starfish 65
Spine Curls with Pillow Squeeze 67
Neck Rolls and Chin Tucks 62
Curl Ups 68
Single Leg Stretch 75
Double Knee Fold 73
Hip Rolls 81
Floating Arms 59
Sitting Side Reach 86
Abductor and Adductor Lifts 87 and 89
Roll Downs 84 or 85
The Pelvic Elevator 70
The Dart 58 or 91
The Rest Position 93

Workout Two

Roll Downs 84 or 85
The Corkscrew 125
Oblique Curl Ups 69
Emergency Stop 71
The Hundred 78
Arm Openings 137
The Dart 58 or 91
Torpedo 90
Front Leg Pull 92
The Rest Position 93

Workout Three

Shoulder Drops 66
Pelvic Stability: Knee Drops and Turn Outs 54
Spine Curls with Pillow Squeeze 67
Hip Flexor Stretch 72
Curl Ups 68
Single Leg Stretch 75 or 76
Hip Rolls 81 or 82
Abductor and Adductor Lifts 87 and 89
The Pelvic Elevator 70
The Diamond Press 107
The Rest Position 93
Scapular Squeeze 160
Roll Downs 84 or 85

Workout Four

The Full Starfish 65
Shoulder Reach 57
Spine Curls with Pillow Squeeze 67
Single Leg Circles 102
Curl Ups 69
The Hundred 78
Hip Rolls 81
Emergency Stop 71
Front Leg Pull 92
Torpedo 90
The Dart 58 or 91
The Rest Position 93

Workout Five

Neck Rolls and Chin Tucks 62
Shoulder Drops 66
Oblique Curl Ups 68
Single Leg Stretch 75
The Pelvic Elevator 70
Arm Openings 137
Sitting Side Reach 86
Abductor and Adductor Lifts 87 and 89
Standing Tarzan 157
Roll Downs 84 or 85
The Diamond Press 107
The Rest Position 93

7 The First Trimester (0–12 weeks)

We only recommend Pilates during the first trimester if you have been regularly practising before you became pregnant. If you are new to Pilates, you should wait until your pregnancy is well established at 16 weeks. Please see page 38.

What's Happening to Your Body?

Just 7–10 days after fertilization the fertilized ovum implants in the uterus. The hormonal changes that take place will have a profound effect on how you feel. Probably the first sign you will have that you are pregnant is that your monthly period is late. You may also notice a change in your breasts quite early on: the nipples become more sensitive and they may tingle and change colour. You might also feel nauseous due to hormonal changes. This could be just in the mornings and may or may not be accompanied by vomiting, but it can happen at any time of the day. Sometimes eating dry biscuits can help.

Now that you are pregnant, you will have to change the way you work out. If you are suffering from morning sickness then you will need to do your workout in the afternoons or evenings. Rest is very important in this first trimester. Be kind to yourself – if you need an afternoon nap, have one.

As your uterus grows it will put pressure on your bladder, so you may feel the need to urinate more frequently. The hormone progesterone also affects your bowels making them more relaxed and sluggish, which means that more water than usual is absorbed. To avoid constipation you must drink extra water and include plenty of fresh fruit and vegetables in your diet. The good news is that by keeping your body moving you are helping to keep your bowels moving! By adding pelvic floor exercises to each session you will improve the circulation in the pelvic area, which will help prevent piles.

You may feel very tired and, as hormones affect your balance and hand to eye coordination, you may feel quite clumsy. You are probably going to feel emotional – think PMT times one hundred. So this is one time you may forgive yourself for crying over the spilt milk! Do not push yourself too hard trying to do everything. Keep your workouts simple and uncomplicated and do not attempt any challenging new exercises.

Your blood pressure will alter. The usual pattern is for a decrease in blood pressure in the first trimester, reaching its lowest midway in your pregnancy, then rising gradually and returning to normal six weeks after the birth. Your antenatal clinic will be keeping a close check on your blood pressure throughout your pregnancy. You may find that exercises such as Roll Downs (pages 84 and 85) make you feel dizzy – if so, leave them out. Give yourself plenty of time to change positions: rolling on to your side as you come up from lying, for example.

It is unlikely that you will put on much weight in the first few weeks, just a few pounds mainly around your waist, which will thicken slightly. You need to accept that your figure is going to change and that pregnancy is not the time to be aiming for a flat stomach – the baby needs room to grow. With this in mind, you should not attempt the more advanced versions of the abdominal exercises. Most Pilates exercises have variations which leave the head down rather than curling it up, for example, Single Leg Stretch (pages 75 and 76). You can still do simple Curl Ups (page 68) and Oblique Curl Ups (page 69), but they should be done slowly and carefully.

In the first chapter, we discussed how hormonal changes affect the ligaments throughout the body making them more like lycra than cotton and thus making your joints more prone to instability. Although your pelvis will be at its most unstable during months 4 to 7, you should take great care when exercising from the onset of your pregnancy. You will need to avoid exercises that have a wide range of movement. From now on, keep your limbs close to your bodyline rather than allowing them to sweep wide. Where appropriate, you may bend the knees rather than having a fully extended leg. For example, when doing Single Leg Circles (page 102), keep the circles small and bend the knee a little. Avoid exercises which place a strain on the pubis symphysis – such as sitting or standing with the legs wide and bending forward.

Let's look a little more closely at the pelvis. If you study the diagram below, you will notice two important ligaments that contribute to its stability: the sacrotuberous ligament attaches to the biceps femoris, one of the hamstring muscles which run down the back of your thighs; the sacrospinous ligament is a lateral stabilizer of the sacrum and has attachments to the pelvic floor and the adductors, the inner-thigh muscles. Because both these ligaments become lax when you are pregnant, the sacroiliac joint becomes vulnerable to injury and less stable. As a result, your hamstring and adductor muscles take on a stabilizing role during pregnancy and post-natally. For this reason, you have to be careful not to overstretch these muscles. If anything, we can focus on strengthening them with exercises like Single Leg Kicks (page 108) and The Pillow Squeeze (page 127).

Remember, too, that your spine will be more prone to hypermobility (too much movement between vertebrae) and that as your breasts become heavier, your thoracic spine may become more rounded, which places a strain on your whole shoulder girdle. Pay close attention to good postural alignment all the time, not just during your sessions. You will need to strengthen your mid-back muscles, so include plenty of scapular stability work and make the most of exercises in which you lie on your front – it's your last chance!

By the end of this first trimester, the baby is already 6 to 7 centimetres (2.5 to 3 inches) long and weighs approximately 45 to 50 grams (2 ounces). It is about the size of an apple and has a beating heart; it can kick, turn its head and swallow.

The risk of miscarriage is greatest during the first trimester and up to 16 weeks into your pregnancy. Please see 'When to Stop Exercising' on page 23.

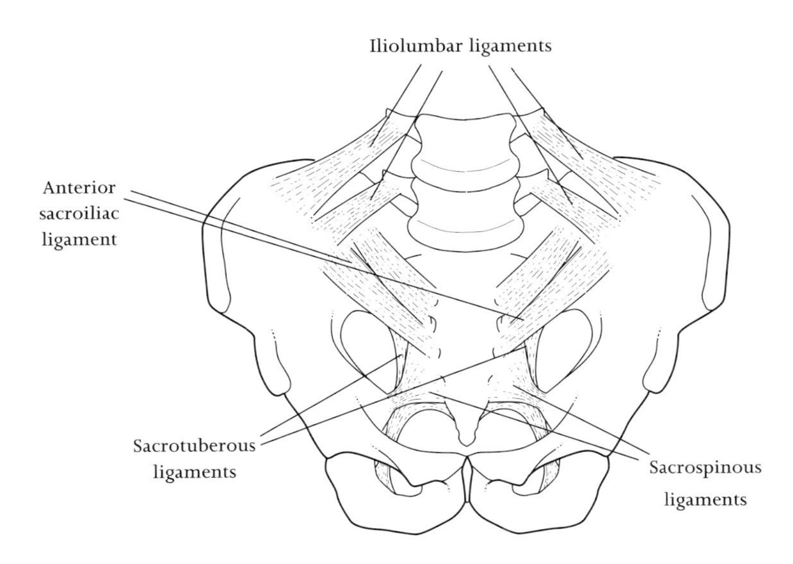

Strong ligaments hold the pelvic bones in place

Guidelines for Exercise in the First Trimester

- Be flexible about the timing of your workout. You cannot exercise if you are feeling nauseous or tired.
- Keep your workouts short and simple.
- Keep the area you are exercising in clear and uncluttered.
- If you are wearing socks, they should be non-slip.
- Do not attempt challenging new exercises – other than the ones we have recommended, which have been specifically chosen.
- Take extra time when moving from one exercise to the next – roll on to your side and wait a moment before rising.
- You may feel dizzy doing Roll Downs (if so, leave them out or you could try the wall version for extra security on page 84).
- Pay close attention to your alignment; do fewer repetitions well rather than lots carelessly.
- Keep your limbs close to your bodyline; bend your knees if you need to when the legs are extended, and keep your range of movement smaller than you would normally.
- Avoid holding stretches for long periods of time.
- Avoid hamstring and adductor stretches – instead, include exercises to strengthen these muscles.
- Do pelvic floor exercises every day.
- You may continue with trunk flexion (Curl Ups) at this stage, but you should do the beginner's versions of the more challenging abdominal exercises such as Single Leg Stretch (page 75).

Recommended Exercises for the First Trimester

Demi Pliés in Turn Out

A lot of Pilates exercises have a ballet influence – they are great for building muscle into the body, especially on the inner thighs and buttocks.

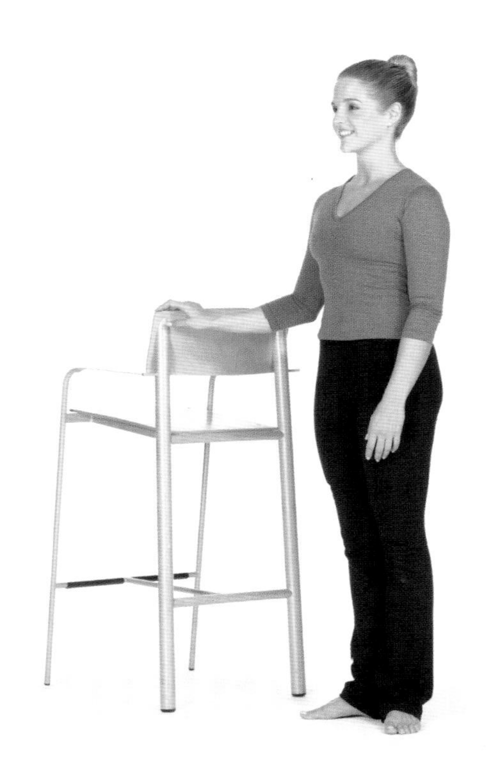

Aim
To learn good postural alignment and to strengthen the inner thighs and buttocks.

Starting Position
Stand tall, side on to the wall or a chair; hold on to the wall or chair. Turn your legs out from the hip joints. It's very important that you do not just turn them out from the knees or ankles – the action comes from the hips. Remember how you turned out the leg in Pelvic Stability (page 56).

Action
1. Breathe in wide and lengthen through the spine.
2. Breathe out, zip up and hollow and stay zipped and hollowed throughout. Bend the knees over the centre of the toes. Keep the heels down and try not to tip forward.
3. Breathe in and slowly straighten your legs, pulling up through the inner thighs and squeezing the buttocks. Feel that you are turning out from deep in the hips.
4. Repeat 8 times.

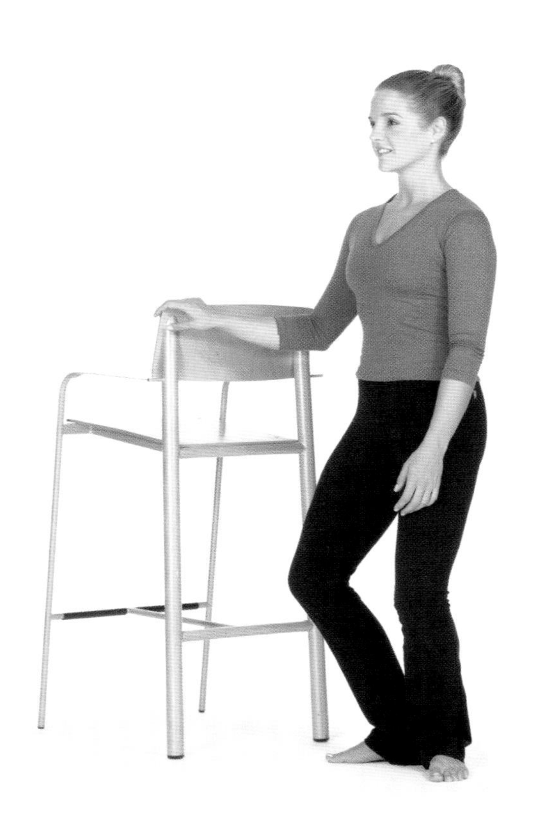

Watchpoints
- Keep good alignment through the body, remember the three main weights of the body – the head, ribcage and pelvis – they should remain balanced over each other.
- Do not stick your bottom out!
- Use your core muscles to keep you centred.
- Feel as though you are being pulled up right through your body from your heels, up the inner thighs through the spine and through the top of the head.

The Dumb Waiter

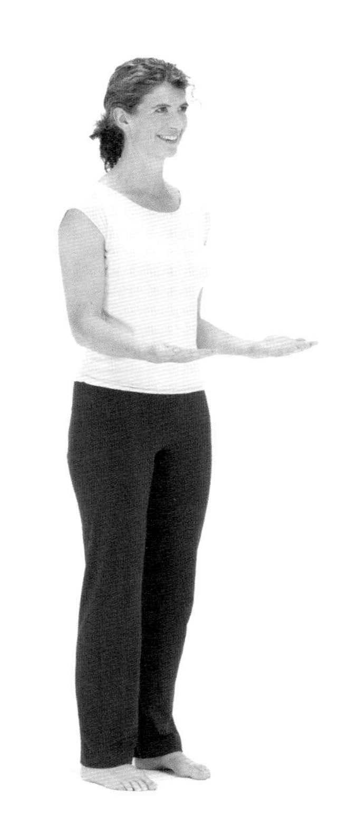

Aim

To become aware of the shoulder blades and of their relationship with the ribcage. To open the chest, especially the front of the upper arms and shoulders. To strengthen the muscles between the shoulder blades.

Equipment

A sturdy chair (optional).

Starting Position

You may sit on a chair or stand for this exercise. If you choose to use the chair, sit well forward with your pelvis in neutral, your feet planted on the floor hip-width apart and your weight even on both buttocks! Bend your arms so your fingers point, palms facing upwards and your elbows tucked into your waist.

Action

1. Breathe in to prepare and lengthen up through the spine.
2. Breathe out, zip up and hollow and stay zipped and hollowed throughout.
3. Breathe in and, keeping your elbows into your sides, move your hands backwards. Work the muscles between the shoulder blades. Keep the shoulder blades down.
4. Breathe out and return the hands to the Starting Position.
5. Repeat 5 times.

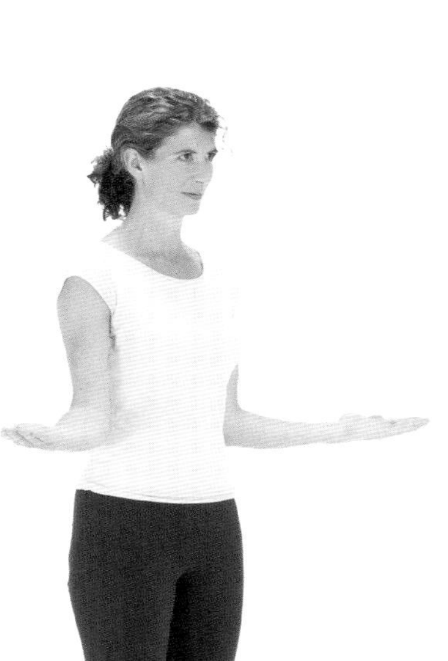

Watchpoints

- Do not allow the upper back to arch as you take the arms back.
- If you find this very easy, check that your elbows are staying in and your shoulder blades stay down.
- Keep your neck released.

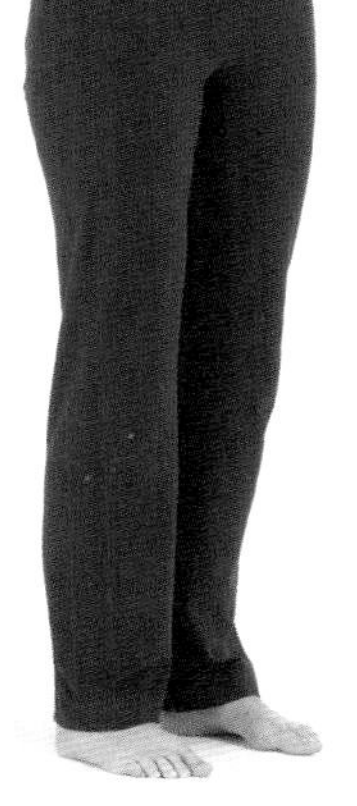

Single Leg Circles

Aim

A classical Pilates exercise which tones the thighs, buttocks and the muscles around the hips. It also mobilizes the hips. You need to use your deep girdle of strength to steady your torso, which means that it is an abdominal exercise as well!

Starting Position

Lie in the Relaxation Position (page 26). Throughout the exercise, you will need to stay aware of what is happening to your torso while the leg moves.

NOTE

Because of the hormonal changes occurring in your body, please keep the leg in the air slightly bent and keep the circles small.

Action (beginner)

1. Breathe in wide to prepare and lengthen through the spine.
2. Breathe out, zip up and hollow and stay zipped throughout. Bend your right leg in, remembering what you learnt in Knee Folds (pages 73 and 74).
3. Breathe in, then as you breathe out slowly straighten the right leg into the air to 90°, if you can, keeping the knee slightly bent.
4. You are now going to circle the leg from the hip joint, first moving it across the body then taking it around outwards and back to the Starting Position.
5. Keep the circles small (about the size of a grapefruit). The idea is that the pelvis and the rest of your body stay still and anchored. You are going to breathe in as you circle across the body, out as you circle away and back towards you.
6. Use your full girdle of strength to keep the body anchored and still. Stay zipped and set the shoulder blades into the back. You may press your shoulder blades into the floor. Your arms will naturally help you to stay stable, but do not rely on them to keep you still – use your core muscles.
7. Repeat 5 circles each way with each leg.

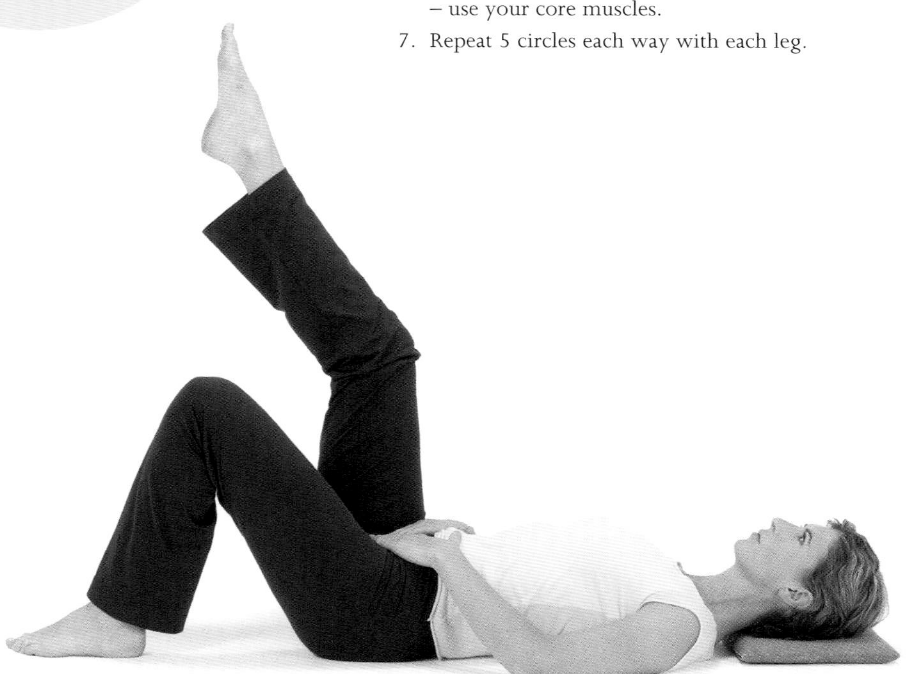

Action (intermediate)

As above, but the leg on the floor is straight. The leg in the air remains slightly bent!

Watchpoints

- Move the leg from the hip joint itself.
- The pelvis stays still and in neutral.
- Keep checking that there is no unnecessary tension in the upper body.

IMPORTANT NOTE

You will need to change position regularly every 3 minutes if you are in your last two trimesters.

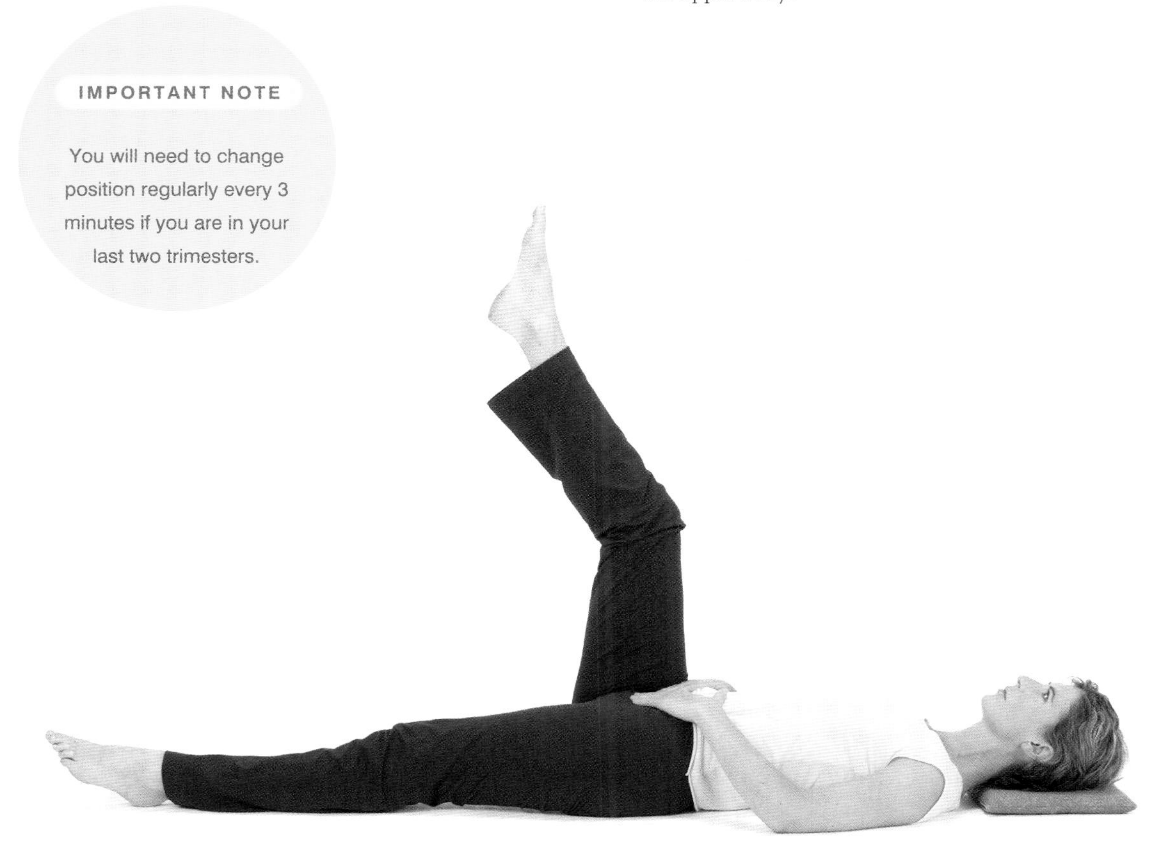

Arm Circles with Weights

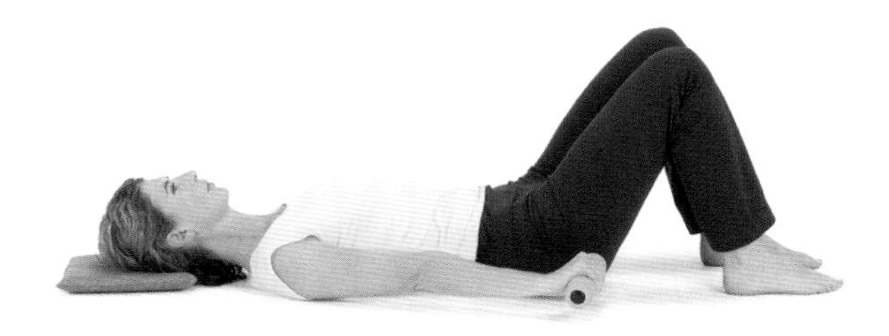

Aim

A great exercise to strengthen the arms and shoulders.

Try it first without the weights to perfect your technique.

Equipment

Hand-held weights of 0.5 kilo (1 pound) each weight.

Starting Position

Lie in the Relaxation Position (page 26). Have your arms down by your sides, with your palms facing down.

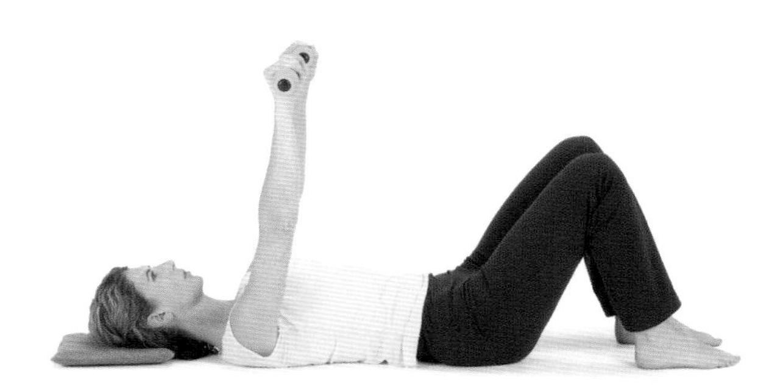

Action

1. Breathe in wide and full. Lengthen through the body.
2. Breathe out, zip up and hollow and stay zipped and hollowed throughout. Raise your arms up and take them behind you.
3. Breathe in as you circle them out to the sides and back down to your body. Turn the palms down as you come back to the starting point.
4. Repeat 5 times, then reverse the direction of the circle and repeat another 5 times.

Watchpoints

- Maintain neutral pelvis and neutral spine throughout and do not allow the upper back to arch.
- Do not allow the ribs to flare. Move with the breath.
- Keep the shoulder blades wide and down the back, but do allow for mobility, no gripping!
- Keep the neck long and released.
- Watch the alignment of the hands and wrists!
- Keep the elbows soft.

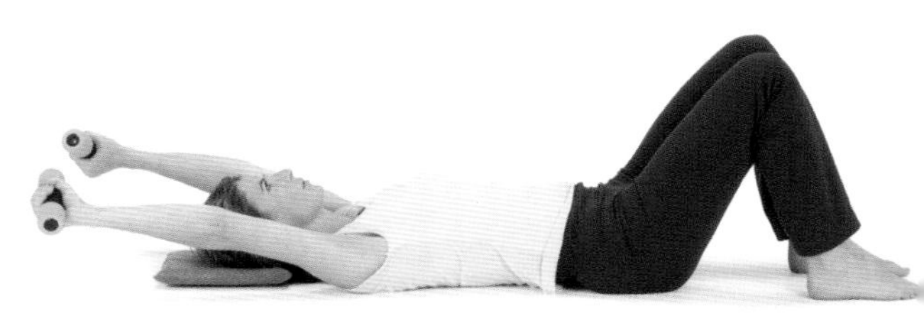

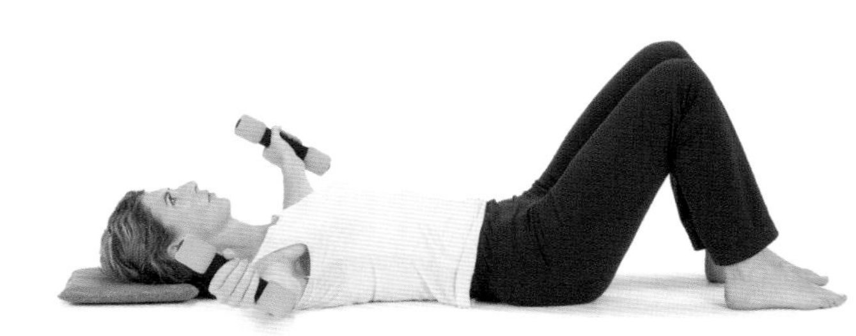

The Star

This exercise has been broken down into two stages.

Aim

To learn how to work from a strong, stable centre.
To work the deep gluteal and the upper back muscles.

NOTE

Avoid this exercise if you are uncomfortable lying on your stomach.

Starting Position: Stage One

Lie on your front with your feet hip-width apart and turned out from the hips. Rest your forehead on your folded arms. Or you can rest your forehead on a flat cushion and place your fingertips on the top of your pelvic bones (this is to check for unwanted movement).

Action

1. Breathe in to prepare and lengthen through the spine.
2. Breathe out and zip up and hollow. Lengthen first, then raise the left leg lifting it no more than 5 centimetres (2 inches) off the ground. Lengthen away from a strong centre. Do not twist in the pelvis; both hip joints stay on the floor. Try to keep your shoulders relaxed and a sense of width in your upper body.
3. Breathe in and relax.
4. Repeat with the other leg.
5. Repeat 5 times with each leg.

Watchpoints

- Keep the lower abdominals supporting your lower back.
- Think of creating space around the hip joint as you lengthen the leg away.
- Be careful to keep both hip joints on the floor – you are only lifting the leg.
- Don't let the pelvis roll or twist, keep it square.
- Keep your neck long and relaxed. The head stays down on the floor throughout the exercise.
- Everyone tries to lift the legs too high, so aim to lift it just a few centimetres.

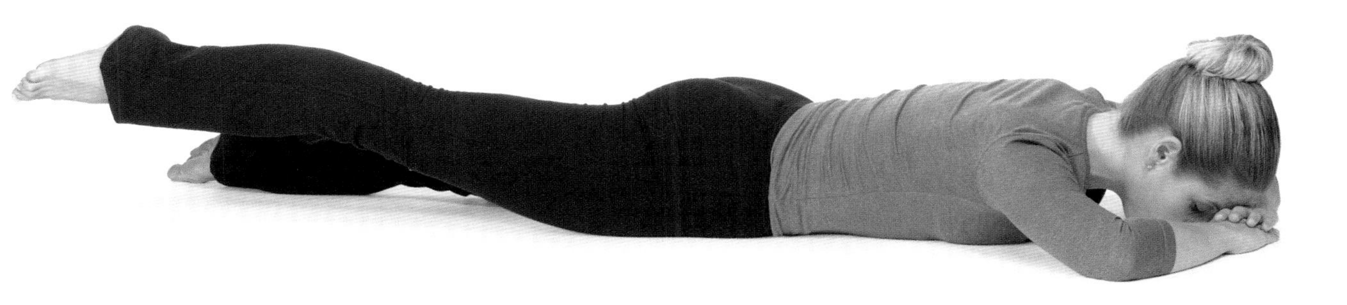

Equipment

A flat cushion.

Starting Position: Stage Two

Lie on your front with your feet hip-width apart and turned out from the hips. Take your arms out above your head just wider than shoulder width so you look like a star, but remember to leave your shoulder blades set down in your back. You may like to place a small, very flat cushion or folded towel under your forehead. The cushion should not alter the angle of your neck.

Action

1. Breathe in to prepare and lengthen through the spine.
2. Breathe out, zip up and hollow, and lengthen. Raise the opposite arm and leg no more than 5 centimetres (2 inches) off the ground. Lengthen away from a strong centre. Do not twist in the pelvis; both hip joints stay on the floor. Try to keep a sense of width in your upper body.
3. Breathe in and relax.
4. Repeat with the other arm and leg.
5. Repeat 5 times to each side.

Watchpoints

- As for Stage One.
- Do not overreach or over-lift the arms. Keep the elbows slightly bent and keep them wide.
- Keep your neck long and relaxed. The head stays down on the floor throughout the exercise.

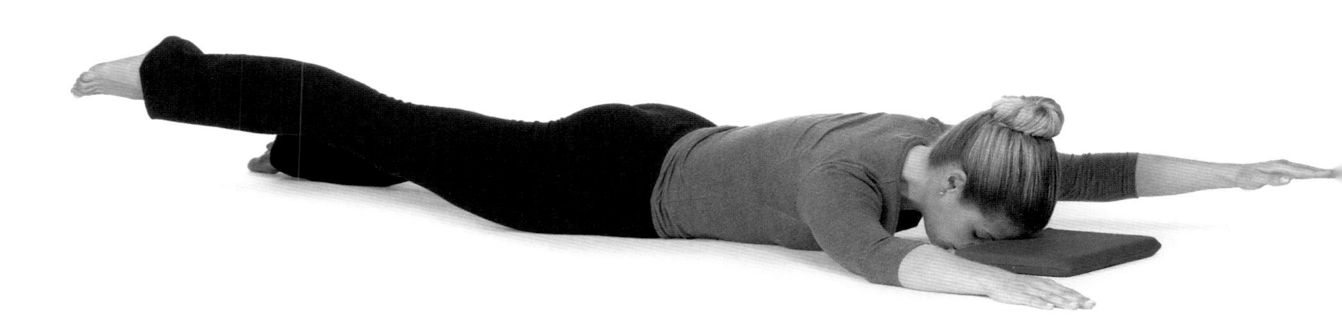

The Diamond Press

You can continue with exercises lying on your front for as long as you are comfortable in this position.

Aim
A subtle exercise, which has dramatic results. It really does help to reverse the effects of being hunched over all day. You can feel the tension in your neck release as the mid-back muscles, which stabilize the shoulder blades, slide down into the back.

Starting Position
Lie on your front with your feet hip-width apart and parallel. Create a diamond shape with your arms by placing your fingertips together just above your forehead. Your elbows are open, your shoulder blades relaxed.

Action

1. Breathe in and lengthen through the spine.
2. Breathe out, zip up and hollow and stay zipped and hollowed throughout. Leading from the crown of the head, bring the head and neck up to neutral, then slide the shoulder blades down into the back of your waist, simultaneously tucking your chin in (as if to hold a ripe peach), and extending your upper body 3 or 4 centimetres (1 or 2 inches) off the floor. Stay looking down at the floor; the back of the neck is long. Imagine a cord pulling you from the top of your head. Really make the connection down into the small of your back – you have to push a little on the elbows, to come up, but this isn't a push-up; make the back muscles work.
3. Breathe in and hold the position. Keep the lower stomach lifted, but the ribs stay on the floor.
4. Breathe out, and slowly lower back down. Keep lengthening through the spine.
5. Repeat 5 times.

Watchpoints

- Keep the lower abdominals drawing back to the spine.
- Make sure you keep looking down at the floor – if you lift your head back you will shorten the back of your neck.
- Really enjoy the sense of your neck growing out from between the shoulder blades.

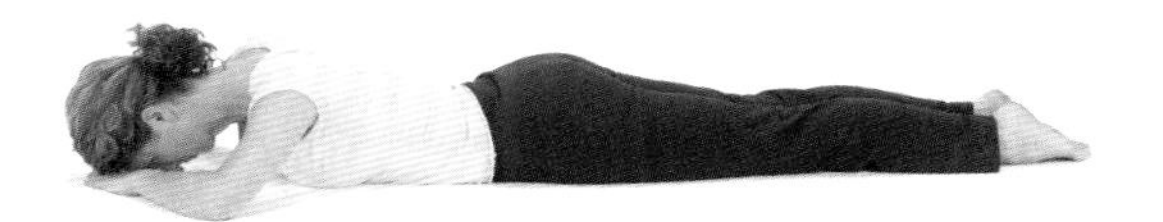

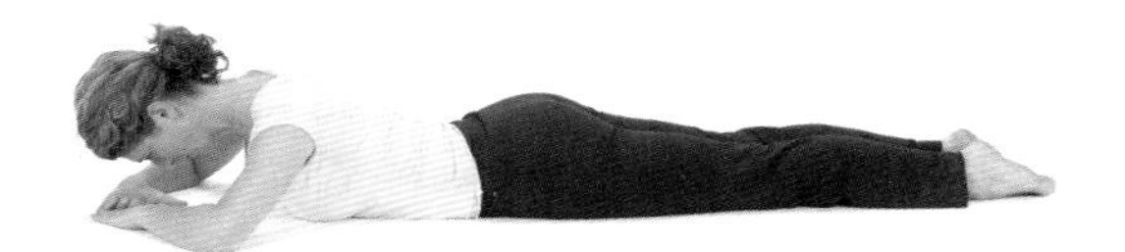

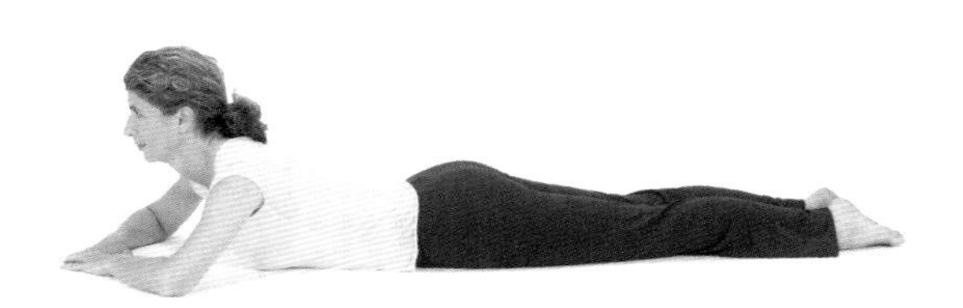

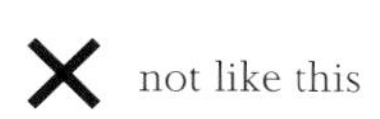

not like this

Single Leg Kicks

Aim
To improve co-ordination. To gently stretch the quadriceps and strengthen the hamstrings. To mobilize the ankle joints.

This exercise can be carried out either in a sphinx position, that is with the upper back extended, or with the head down, resting on the folded hands. You should be comfortable with the Diamond Press (page 107) and Dart (page 91) before you attempt to extend the back further.

Starting Position
If you are coming up into a sphinx position, place the hands on the floor just wider than shoulder-width apart, so the fingers are in line with your ears. Zip up and hollow. Lengthen through the crown of the head and let it lead the movement as you push down on to the forearms; bring your shoulder blades down into your back and raise the upper body off the floor. The elbows stay down. Make sure your neck remains long and the shoulders stay well away from the ears and the breastbone. Your pelvis and pubic bone remain on the floor. The navel is lifted to the spine throughout the exercise. You should feel comfortable in this position. If you feel any pinching in your back, come down to the alternative position.

In the alternative position, rest your forehead on your folded hands. Make sure that your upper back remains open and relaxed.

Action
1. With the legs slightly apart, zip up and hollow and pulse the right foot into the buttocks, keeping the foot pointed. Fold the foot in 3 times pointed and 3 times flexed.
2. Repeat with the other foot.
3. Breathe normally throughout the exercise.
4. Repeat 3 times with each leg.
5. Follow this exercise with the Rest Position on page 93.

Watchpoints
- If you are in the sphinx position, do not allow yourself to sink down, keep lengthening and zipping up and hollowing.
- In either position, make sure that both hips stay in balanced contact with the floor.
- Maintain the distance between the ears and the shoulders.
- Keep pushing gently into the floor to work the upper arms.
- Do not allow your back to collapse.

NOTE

Take advice if you have a back or knee injury.

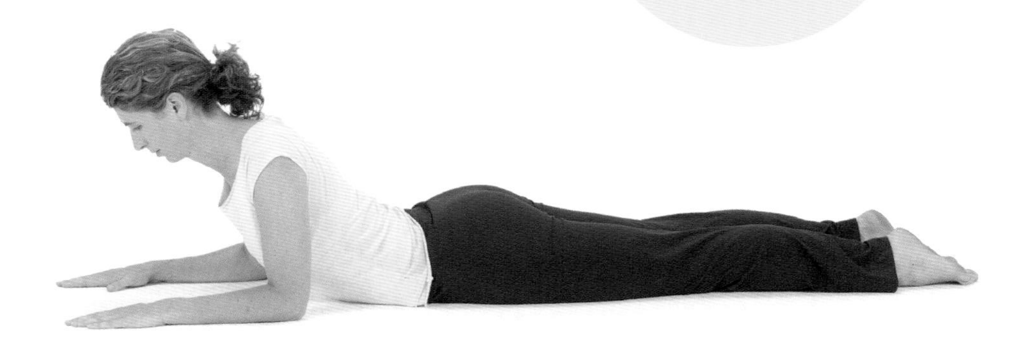

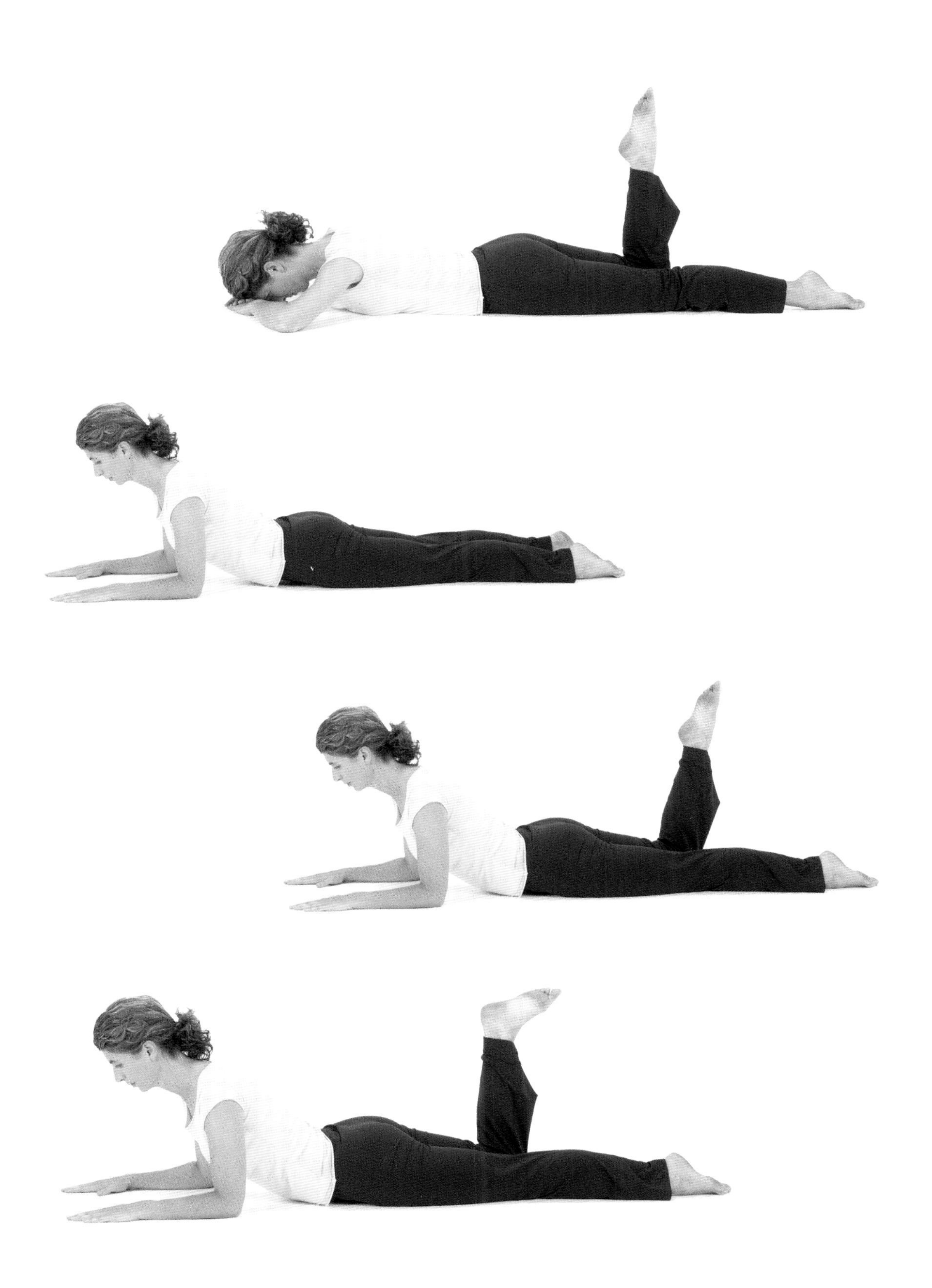

Threading a Needle

Aim
To relax the upper back, especially the muscles between the shoulders.

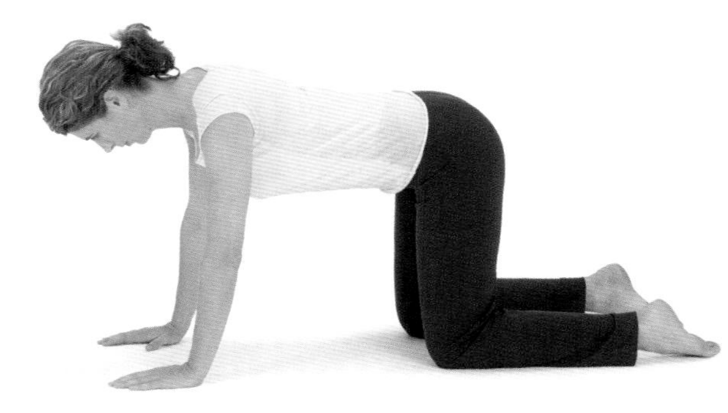

Starting Position
Come on to all fours with the hands under the shoulders and the knees under the hips. Have a long neck and the head in good alignment with the spine. You will be looking straight down at the floor.

Action
1. Breathe in wide and full, and transfer your weight on to your left hand.
2. Breathe out, zip up and hollow, and lift your right hand off and put the back of it on the floor. The elbow is open.
3. Slide the back of the right hand along the mat under the right arm. The elbow has to bend. Keep both shoulders down into the back. The head moves naturally with the movement in line with the spine.
4. Breathe in and stay in this position.
5. Breathe out and return to the starting point.
6. Repeat 3 times on each arm.
7. Follow this with the Rest Position on page 93.

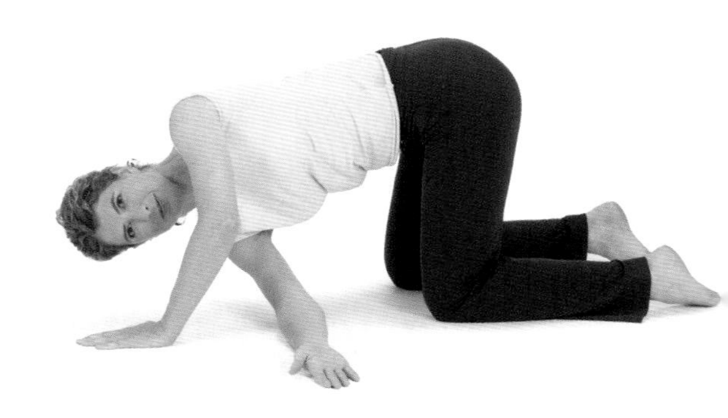

Watchpoints
- Keep lengthening through the spine.
- Try not to stick your bottom out too far!
- You may rest the side of your head on the floor if you wish.

The Big Squeeze

Aim
To work the muscles of the lower abdomen, pelvic floor, the buttocks and the inner thighs, keeping the upper body relaxed.

Equipment
A small cushion.

Starting Position
Lie on your front. Place, or get a close friend to, a small cushion between the tops of your thighs. Rest your forehead on your folded hands; open and relax the shoulders.

Have your toes together and your heels apart.

Action
1. Breathe in wide and full to prepare and lengthen through the spine.
2. Breathe out. Zip up from the pelvic floor and hollow the lower abdominals up to the spine as if there is a fragile egg under the stomach and you do not wish to crush it.
3. Tighten the buttocks, squeeze the inner thighs and the cushion, and bring the heels together! Hold for a count of 5. Keep breathing normally and check continuously that you are only working from the waist down. Then release. Keep your feet on the floor.
4. Repeat the Big Squeeze 5 times.
5. Come into the Rest Position on page 93.

Watchpoints
- Keep your neck and jaw relaxed as you squeeze.
- Feel the full length of your body from the top of your head to the tips of your toes.
- Feel you buttocks and upper thighs wrapping round the cushion.

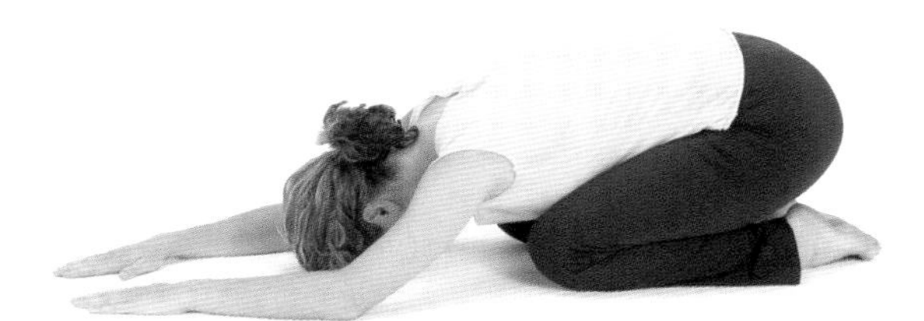

Rest position

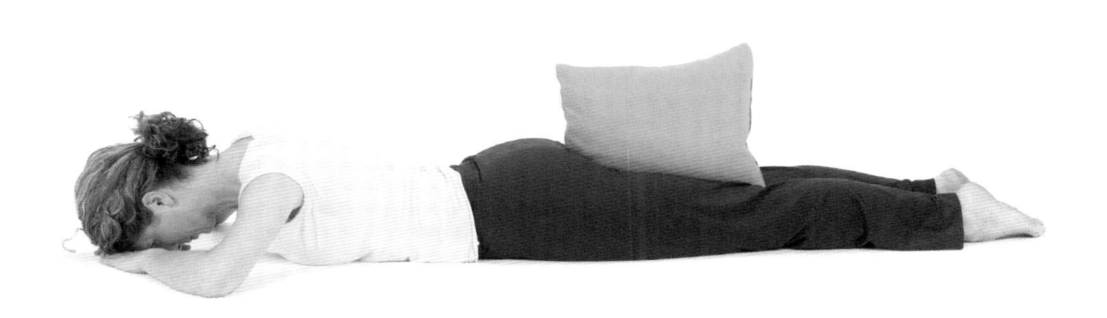

Ankle Circles

This exercise can also be done sitting on a chair. You will need to support the working leg by holding it behind the thigh just above the knee, or you can place a rolled-up towel there. It is a wonderful way to help reduce swelling in the feet and ankles.

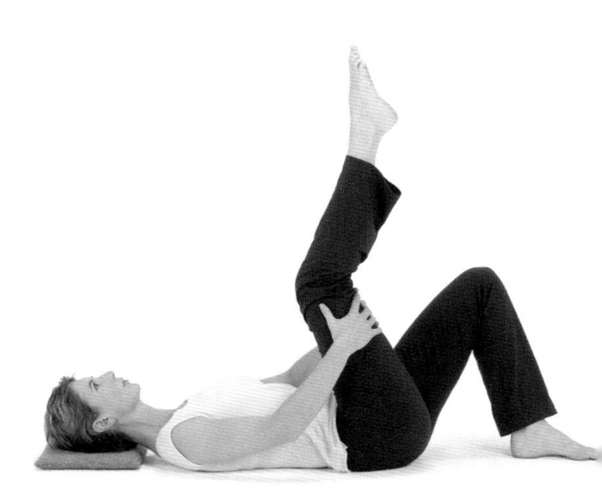

Aim
To free the ankle joint, increasing its mobility. To work the muscles, ligaments and tendons surrounding the ankle joint. To work the calf muscles.

Equipment
A chair and a towel (optional).

Starting Position
Lie on your back in the Relaxation Position (page 26) or sit on a chair. Bend one knee up and take hold of it just behind the knee, with your thumbs coming round in front of the knee – this is so that you can feel if your leg is moving.

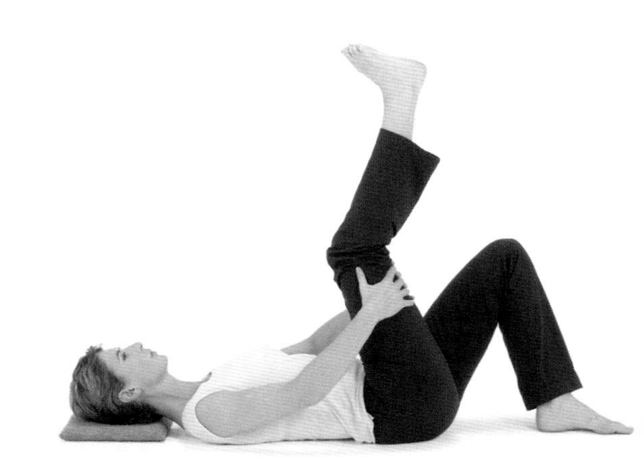

Action
1. Slowly start to circle the foot around very, very slowly and, taking it as far as you can, go to the maximum. The leg should stay completely still, the movement comes totally from the ankle joint. Do not just wiggle your toes around.
2. Do 5 circles each way.

Watchpoints
- What was happening to the rest of your body?
- Remember, shoulder blades down, breastbone soft, elbows open, lateral breathing, neutral pelvis.
- You do not need to zip up and hollow throughout this exercise, so use this as a break from stabilizing.

First Trimester Workouts

There are 5 balanced workouts set out below. Each lasts approximately 20–30 minutes, and you should try to do all 5 workouts once each week.

The exercises are mainly drawn from this chapter but we have also added a few from earlier and later chapters which will make the workouts more varied. You can of course add any exercise from later in the book if you wish.

Work at whichever level you feel comfortable with, moving on to stage or level two of an exercise (where applicable) when you feel ready, unless a level is recommended in the listing. For example, Hip Rolls (Level One only); this exercise **must** be done with the feet on the ground throughout pregnancy.

Workout One

Pelvic Stability: Knee Folds and Drops 55
Baby Spine Curls with Pillow Squeeze 123
Neck Rolls and Chin Tucks 62
Curl Ups (just 5 repetitions) 68
Single Leg Stretch (Level One only) 75
Hip Rolls (Level One only) 81
The Pelvic Elevator 70
Demi Pliés in Turn Out 100
Sitting Side Reach 86
The Star 105 and 106
The Rest Position 93

Workout Two

Dumb Waiter 101
Roll Downs Against the Wall 84
The Corkscrew 125
Single Leg Circles 102
Oblique Curl Ups (just 6 repetitions) 69
Arm Circles (With or Without Weights) 104
Ankle Circles 112
The Pelvic Elevator 70 / Emergency Stop 71
Single Leg Kicks 108
Threading a Needle 110
The Big Squeeze 111
The Diamond Press 107
The Rest Position 93

Workout Three

The Full Starfish 65
Baby Spine Curls with Pillow Squeeze 123
Ankle Circles 112
Curl Ups (5 repetitions) 68
Hip Rolls (Level One only) 81
The Oyster 149
The Pelvic Elevator 70
Roll Downs Against the Wall 84
Sitting Side Reach 86
Back Press 158
Ankle Circles 112
The Star 105 or 106
The Diamond Press 107
The Rest Position 93

Workout Four

Shoulder Drops 66
Neck Rolls and Chin Tucks 62
Single Leg Circles 102
Single Leg Stretch (Level One only) 75
Arm Openings 137
The Pelvic Elevator 70 / Emergency Stop 71
Abductor and Adductor Lifts (no weights) 87 and 89
The Dart 58 or 91
The Big Squeeze 111
Threading a Needle 110
The Rest Position 93
Roll Downs Against the Wall 84

Workout Five

Demi Pliés in Turn Out 100
The Dumb Waiter 101
Baby Spine Curls with Pillow Squeeze 123
Curl Ups (just 5 repetitions) 68
Hip Rolls (Level One only) 81
The Oyster 149
Pelvic Elevator 70
Arm Circles (With or Without Weights) 104
Sitting Side Reach 86
Single Leg Kicks 108
The Big Squeeze 111
The Rest Position 93

8 The Second Trimester (13–26 weeks)

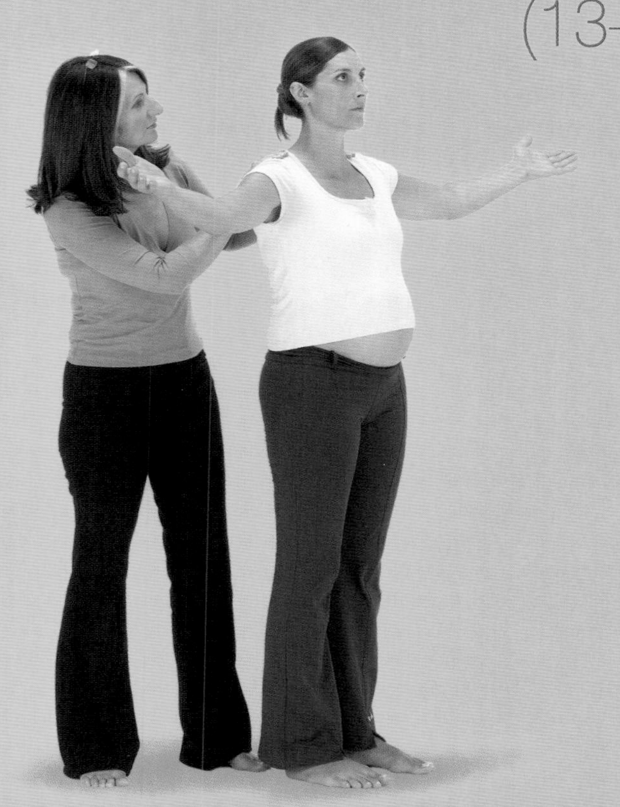

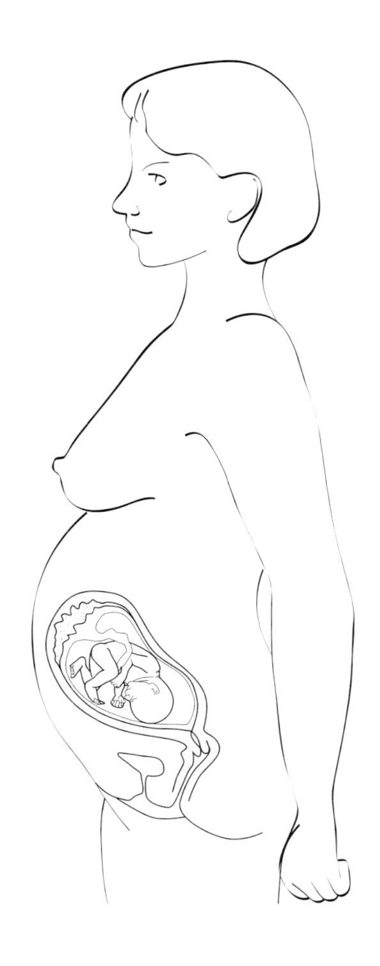

What's Happening to Your Body?

By the second trimester, your pregnancy will begin to show to the outside world. This is the best trimester in terms of how you feel because most women lose the tiredness and nausea of the early stage of pregnancy and feel fantastic; they really 'glow'. This isn't always the case, however, and unfortunately some mothers continue to feel tired, especially if they have young children to run around after!

It is around the 20-week mark that you first feel the baby move inside you; this is called the quickening, and is a truly magical moment. By the end of this trimester, the baby will be approximately 30 centimetres (12 inches) in length, weigh 900 grams (2.5 pounds approx.), and will have eyebrows, eyelashes and fingernails. The baby will be flexing its own muscles and may well be experimenting with its own fitness techniques such as somersaulting, football and cycling, though by far the strangest feeling of all is when it gets the hiccups!

It is now even more essential that you plan regular Pilates sessions into your schedule. If you are still working this may prove difficult, but even short sessions will ultimately pay off. You may still feel rather clumsy, because the changes in your hormones affect your spatial awareness and hand to eye co-ordination. It will also become increasingly difficult for you to see your feet, so make sure the area where you are exercising is clear. For the same reasons, take extra care if you are using weights or other equipment. Keep your workouts simple and do fewer repetitions of each exercise than normal.

Obviously, as the baby grows it is going to be increasingly difficult for you to exercise on your front. You can continue with front-lying exercises quite safely until you feel uncomfortable in this position. As most Pilates back extension exercises (for example the Dart on page 91) involve lying on your front, you will need to find other ways to perform this movement, such as the gentle Chest Expansion on page 131. Take care when doing any back extension that you extend only the upper back and do not take the stretch into the low back.

Quite naturally your appetite will increase, but so too does your tendency to flatulence, bloating, heartburn and indigestion! You will need to plan the timing of your workouts accordingly. It is not advisable to exercise on an empty stomach, but neither should you exercise on a full one or you may find yourself burping, or worse, throughout the session! Eat something light, perhaps a couple of hours beforehand to sustain you. If you normally work out in the evening, bear in mind that you should not eat a heavy meal afterwards late in the evening or indigestion will keep you up all night! You may find that exercises such as Floating Arms (page 59), Arm Circles (page 104) and the Corkscrew (page 125) take the pressure off the diaphragm and help with indigestion.

There may also be some other rather uncomfortable side effects to your pregnancy: you may find your eyesight worsens – a result of the changes in your hormones; you will be more prone to headaches, nasal congestion, nosebleeds and sinus infections. Thankfully, exercise will help to boost your immune system and make you better able to cope with infections. As you learn to identify and release tension throughout the body, you should, hopefully, be able to overcome or prevent tension headaches.

As your uterus grows, your navel starts to protrude and the pigmentation of your skin and the linea alba, which runs from your navel down, will darken in colour. At this stage of your pregnancy, hollowing your lower abdominals back to your spine may sound like an impossible task! Obviously you are not going to get an actual hollow now, but you should still think about zipping up and hollowing because this action gives you stability. Think about lifting your bump as you zip up.

Your breasts will also be growing substantially now. By the end of your pregnancy they may have increased in weight by as much as 900 grams (2.5 pounds approx.). If you haven't already done so, invest in a good bra that supports you well. Think about what happens when old bras lose their support: they tend to ride up at the back. You are going to need good mid-back muscles to keep your upper body in good alignment and to carry the increased weight of your breasts. This is when all the work you have done on scapular stability during the preparatory stage and during your first trimester is going to pay off. But even if you have only just started Pilates in this second trimester, there is still lots that can be done to strengthen these all-important muscles. Exercises like the Corkscrew (page 125) and Windows (page 132) are perfect for this.

We saw in The Importance of Good Posture (page 11) that your centre of gravity is going to alter as your uterus grows. Now is the time to check your posture or ask a friend to help you do so. Your posture will change month by month. If you notice an increased lumbar curve (see page 11) then you should avoid any exercise that takes your lumbar spine further into extension. That means avoiding exercises such as Single Leg Kicks (page 108). You will need to do some upper-body extension – Chest Expansion (page 131) is great, but you must take extra care that you do not arch your lower back. If in doubt, leave it out! On the other hand, Baby Spine Curls (page 123), the Rest Position (page 93) and Sliding Down the Wall: Variation Two (page 136) are perfect for correcting the curve and releasing tension in the low back.

If, however, you have noticed that your back has flattened with your pregnancy and you have swayed back and lost the natural curve in your lumbar spine, you must be very aware when you sit and stand and do the exercises that you keep a neutral spine and pelvis. Variation One of Sliding Down the Wall (page 135) is perfect for you. You can still do Baby Spine Curls (page 123) and the Rest Position (page 93), but take a few extra moments when you recover to find neutral pelvis.

Let's look once more at what happens to the abdominals as your pregnancy develops because this is going to influence which exercises are safe and which are potentially dangerous for your health. Once again, it is inadvisable to assume that every woman is the same; the relative strength of the abdominals is going to vary enormously from mother to mother. For example, a woman who has practised Pilates regularly will have a very strong abdominal wall, which is going to cope far better with the extra size and weight of the uterus. A mother who has never exercised, or who has done the wrong kind of exercises, will naturally have weaker abdominals. Other factors also come into play: previous pregnancies might also have caused a stretch weakness; a previous caesarean section or abdominal surgery may have resulted in weakened abdominals.

By the end of the second trimester, the uterus will be about the size of a basketball. As we discussed in Preparing for Your Pregnancy, to accommodate this growth, the abdominals elongate and the linea alba, the line dividing the six pack, the rectus abdominis, separates. If you have good abdominal tone this is usually not a problem and the two sides will naturally come together in the early weeks after the birth. But with poor abdominal tone the separation can remain significant (see page 180 for the post-natal 'rec' check). Any separation which remains at 2 centimetres (approximately two fingers) is considered a problem. This condition, known as diastasis recti, reduces the ability of the abdominal muscles to control the pelvis and the spine. In severe cases, herniation can occur.

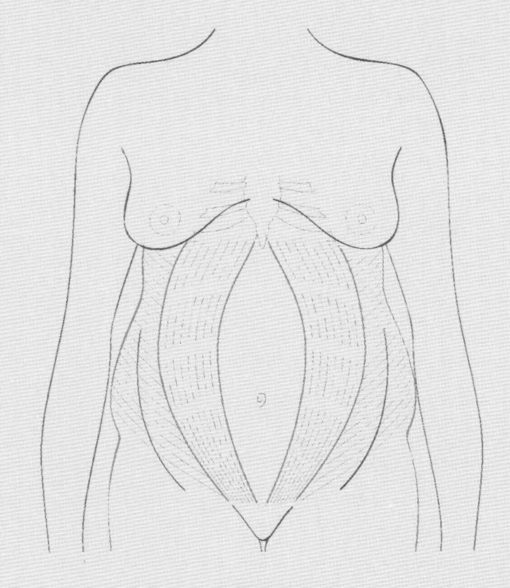

Diastasis recti

Notice how the separation of the rectus abdominis has changed the angle at which the fibres run. This muscle is responsible for trunk flexion (for example curling up from the floor), so with its separation you are going to get a different angle of pull. This is why we do not recommend you do any curl ups or flexion of the trunk from the second trimester onwards. Unfortunately this means that such favourite exercises as Single Leg Stretch, the Hundred and even basic Curl Ups should be avoided. The two sides of the muscle must rejoin before you can restart curl ups otherwise, if you exercise with the separation, you risk strengthening the abdominals in this separated position – apart! However, in Body Control Pilates we have a hundred and one other ways of making you work those abdominals! Besides, we have already seen how it is the deeper corset-like transversus abdominis muscle, which you work with the zip up and hollow, that holds the key to regaining the flatter stomach.

You may find in the later months that fluid accumulation can result in leg cramps. These can happen at any time but are most likely to occur at night after the fluids have collected in the legs all day. Try to avoid standing for long periods and make sure you do not do too many standing exercises in a row. Occasionally, pointing the toes can also cause a leg cramp. If you do get one, the answer is to flex the foot bringing the toes towards your face. We have also given you a Calf Stretch on page 130, which will help relieve the cramps. Otherwise, you can help to prevent them by elevating the legs during the day.

After 16 weeks, you need to be very careful not to lie supine (on your back) for longer than 3 minutes at a time. This can result in a condition known as supine hypotensive syndrome, where the supply of blood to the brain is reduced. When lying flat, the uterus may compress the vena cava and restrict the flow of blood back to the brain. A feeling of light-headedness or dizziness is a symptom. Because many Pilates exercises involve lying on your back, you will need to plan the order in which you do your exercises very carefully and you will also need to time yourself so that after 3 minutes you change position. Normally one set of Leg Slides (page 54), for example, will take you about 3 minutes to complete, but you may need to reduce the number of repetitions. Everyone works at a different pace and the workouts we have given for this trimester take this into account. We recommend that a supine exercise is followed by one lying on your side, or by a sitting exercise before coming back down on the floor. This means a frequent change of position, and you must take the extra time to do this. Remember, too, that this condition isn't restricted to exercise sessions. It can affect you if you have a massage, for example. If you do feel light-headed or nauseous, try lying on your left side.

Remember that this is the trimester when you are most unstable in your joints especially around the pelvis. You must avoid any movements that may put a strain on your sacroiliac joints and your pubis symphysis. For the same reason, you should continue to avoid hamstring and adductor stretches. The recommended exercises in the programme and in the workouts will help to promote pelvic stability without compromising it.

As we discussed earlier, during pregnancy your blood volume is going to increase, and this may have some uncomfortable side effects. Swollen tissue may press on nerves causing neural signs (pins and needles and numbness) in your fingers and toes. This is normal in pregnancy. However, if the numbness and pain are limited to your thumb, index finger, middle finger and half of the fourth finger, then it indicates carpal tunnel syndrome when the carpal tunnel in the wrist becomes swollen resulting in pressure on the nerves which pass through it. Sometimes the discomfort may also affect the hand, wrist and arm. The problem is often particularly troublesome at night because the effects of gravity result in fluids collecting in the hands during the day. Your doctor may suggest wearing splints on your wrists at night to keep your wrist joint in a neutral position, which helps to keep the carpal tunnel open. When exercising, try to do the same, that is to keep good neutral alignment of the shoulders, wrists and hands. Four-point kneeling may prove a problem and aggravate your symptoms. You can try holding a rolled-up towel in your hands or placing a flat cushion or folded towel under the heel of your hands (see photo) to lessen the angle at the wrist.

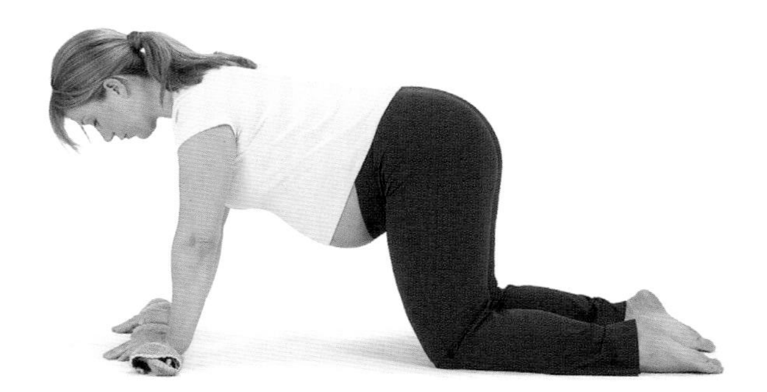

In the first chapter we mentioned how hormonal changes are going to cause the relaxation of the muscle tissue in your veins, and that this, combined with an increase in blood volume, fluid retention, the extra weight gain of pregnancy, the relaxation of the muscle tissue and the added pressure of the uterus on the pelvic area may result in oedema, varicose veins and haemorrhoids. Fortunately, there are lots of Pilates exercises which boost the circulatory and lymphatic systems and help to keep those fluids moving. Exercises such as Walking on the Spot (page 124) and Ankle Circles (page 112) work the deep calf pump and help the valves work efficiently. Pelvic floor exercises will improve circulation to the pelvic area. You can also help by not standing for too long, wearing support tights or socks, avoiding high heels, drinking plenty of water to avoid constipation and thus avoiding straining, and by keeping your weight gain within guidelines. Walking briskly will also help to get the calf pump working.

From this stage in your pregnancy, we will start to add squatting exercises. Squatting opens the pelvic outlet and is a natural birth position because it allows gravity to assist!

NOTE

As your pregnancy progresses you may find it difficult to get down on and up from the floor – see page 144.

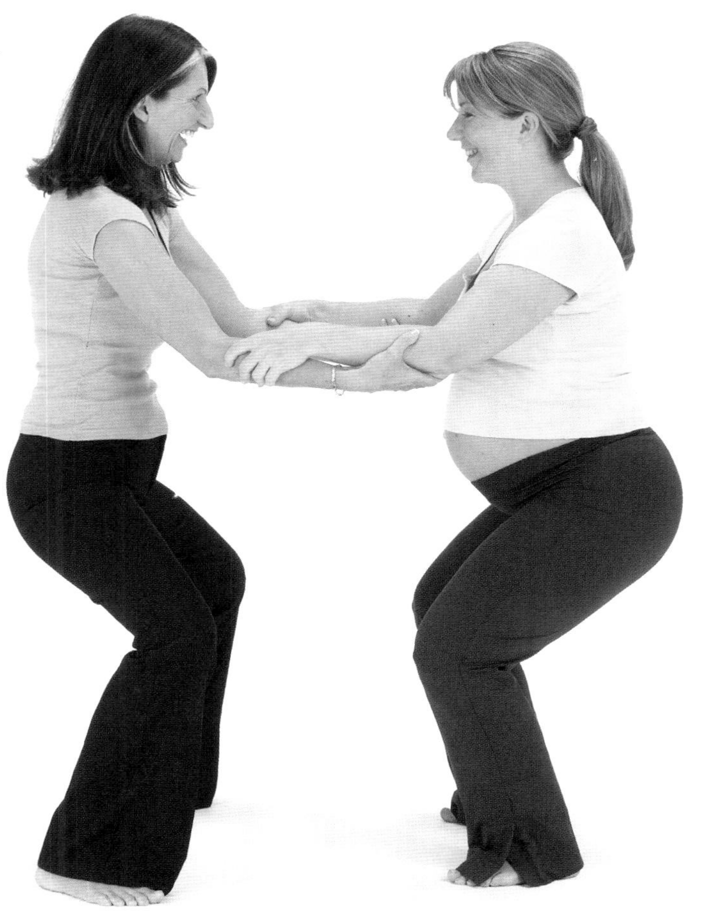

Taking Up Pilates in the Second Trimester

If you are new to Pilates, we advise you to wait until you are at least 16 weeks pregnant before you start the programme. This means you will have to learn the basics and some of the exercises that have been recommended in the chapters on Preparing for Your Pregnancy and The First Trimester.

Bear in mind that by 16 weeks you should avoid lying on your back for longer than 3 minutes, so change position frequently. All the other guidelines for the second trimester will also apply.

Learn the following exercises before starting the second trimester programme:

From Chapter 5: The Basics of Body Control Pilates

- Breathing 45
- The Compass 46
- The Pelvic Elevator 49
- Stabilizing on all Fours 50
- Pelvic Stability: Leg Slides, Knee Drops, Knee Folds and Turn Out. But remember to change position after each one so that you do not stay on your back for longer than 3 minutes. Intersperse these exercises with sitting, standing or front-lying exercises (while you can). 54
- Shoulder Reach 57
- The Dart (Stage One) if you can 58
- Floating Arms 59
- The Starfish (if you can) 61
- Neck Rolls and Chin Tucks 62

From Chapter 6: Preparing for Your Pregnancy

- The Full Starfish 65
- Hip Rolls (Level One only, feet down) 81
- Roll Downs: Rolling Down a Wall 84
- Sitting Side Reach 86
- Abductor Lifts 87
- Adductor Lifts 89
- The Dart (Stage Two) if you can 91
- The Rest Position 93

From Chapter 7: The First Trimester (0–12 weeks)

- Demi Pliés in Turn Out 100
- The Dumb Waiter 101
- Single Leg Circles 102
- Arm Circles with Weights 104
- Threading a Needle 110
- Ankle Circles 112

You are now ready to start the main programme for the second trimester!

Guidelines for Exercising in the Second Trimester

You should:

- Keep sessions to a manageable length so you do not tire.
- Take extra care as you will be a little clumsy.
- Be careful when moving from one position to the next – allow extra time. If coming up from lying, roll on to your side and then wait a moment before rising slowly.
- Do fewer repetitions of each exercise.
- Plan your sessions to take into account meal times and any indigestion you may suffer.
- Do not spend longer than 3 minutes lying on your back; change positions frequently.
- If you feel at all dizzy, lie on your left side – this is also an ideal position for resting.
- Do front-lying exercises for as long as is comfortable, then stop. Try to include some back extensions such as Chest Expansion (page 131) at each workout.
- Continue with the zip up and hollow action even though there is not much in the way of a hollow. Think of lifting your bump. Zip and lift.
- Take a moment to relax between exercises so that your abdominals can have a break.
- Do pelvic floor exercises every session and every day.
- Always include exercises for scapular stability such as the Corkscrew (page 125) and Windows (page 132) to prevent poor posture, in particular to stop you from becoming round shouldered, and to help support the added weight of the breasts.
- Identify how your posture is changing/has changed and choose your exercises accordingly.
- If you have an increased hollow in your low back, then avoid taking extension into this area.
- Avoid any exercise which involves curling up from the mat (flexion), therefore no Curl Ups, Single Leg Stretches, Hundreds, etc.
- Include exercises, Ankle Circles for example on page 112, which elevate the legs and work the calf pump to help improve circulation.
- Include calf stretches to help prevent leg cramps.
- Because of instability around the pelvis, continue to avoid exercises with a wide range of movement and/or long levers. Keep your limbs close to your bodyline and bend the knees when necessary. Do not use leg weights.
- Do hamstring and adductor stretches with caution. Overstretching these muscle groups can increase pelvic instability or hypermobility.
- Avoid exercises which put any pressure on the pubis symphysis. This is liable to separate with the increased laxity of the ligaments. There are no such exercises in this book but you may find them elsewhere, for example the Sitting Wide Leg Stretch.
- Avoid holding any position or stretches for long periods of time.
- Try not to do too many standing positions in a row.
- Take care with balancing or weight-bearing exercises on one leg, as this may promote sacroiliac or pubis symphysis discomfort.
- Consider using a wedge or a rolled-up towel under the sitting bones in sitting exercises.
- Empty your bladder before a workout to save you having to interrupt the session and to avoid mishaps!

Recommended Exercises for the Second Trimester

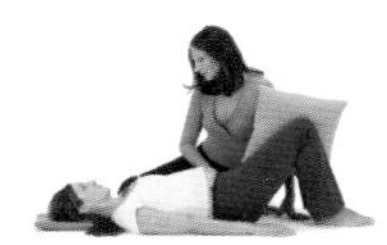

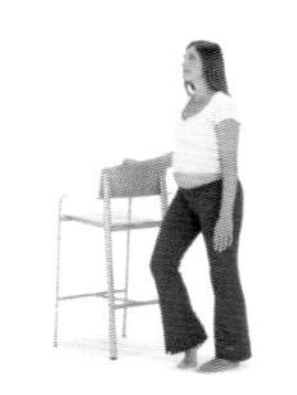

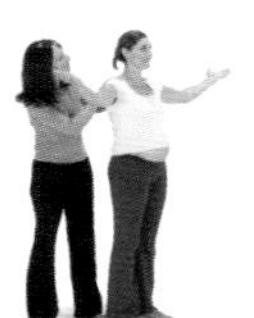

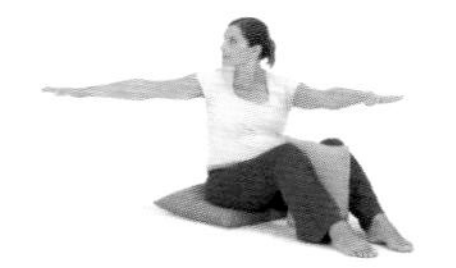

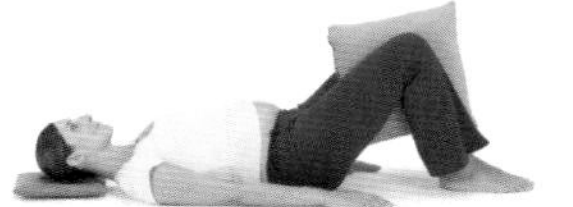

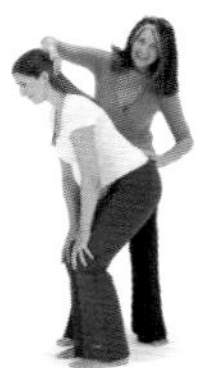

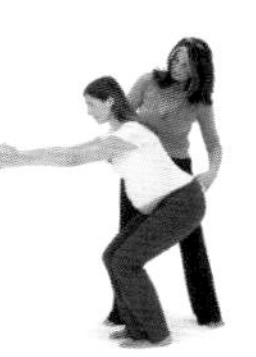

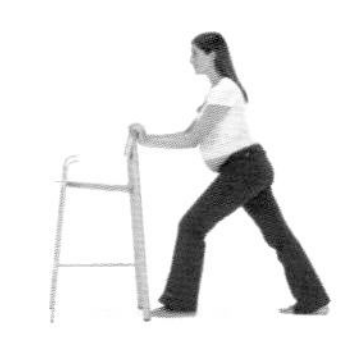

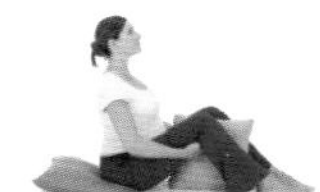

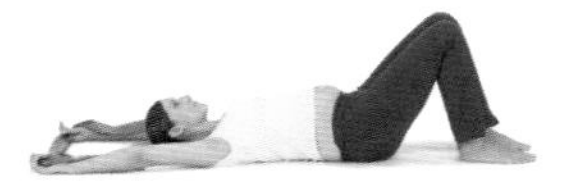

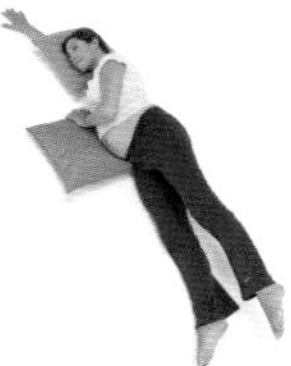

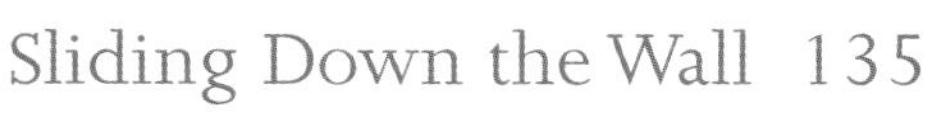

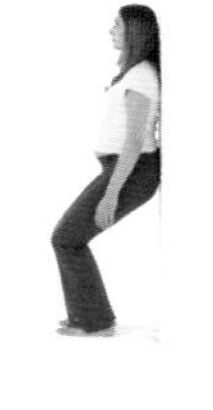

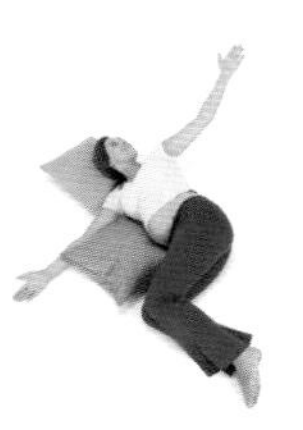

Baby Spine Curls with Pillow Squeeze

Aim
This is a variation on the normal Spine Curls.

Equipment
A plump pillow.

Starting Position
Lie in the Relaxation Position (page 26), checking that your feet are parallel and a few centimetres apart, and about 30 centimetres (12 inches) from your buttocks. Place the pillow between your knees. Your arms are relaxed down by your sides, palms facing down.

With this version, you should not take too much of your spine off the mat. Work within your comfort range. Focus on lengthening the base of the spine and working the pelvic floor, buttocks and inner thighs.

Action
1. Breathe in wide to prepare.
2. Breathe out, zip up and hollow and stay zipped and hollowed throughout. Squeeze the cushion between the knees, squeeze your buttocks and curl the tailbone off the floor just a little.
3. Breathe in, and slowly curl back down to neutral, lengthening out the spine.
4. Breathe out and peel a little more of the spine off the floor; really try to get the base of the spine open.
5. Breathe in and then breathe out, as you place the spine back down, bone by bone.
6. Repeat these Baby Spine Curls up to 6 times. Move the spine on the out-breath.

Watchpoints
- Keep the weight even on both feet and try not to let them roll in or out.
- Keep your neck long and soft.
- Don't curl up too far – it's a small movement.

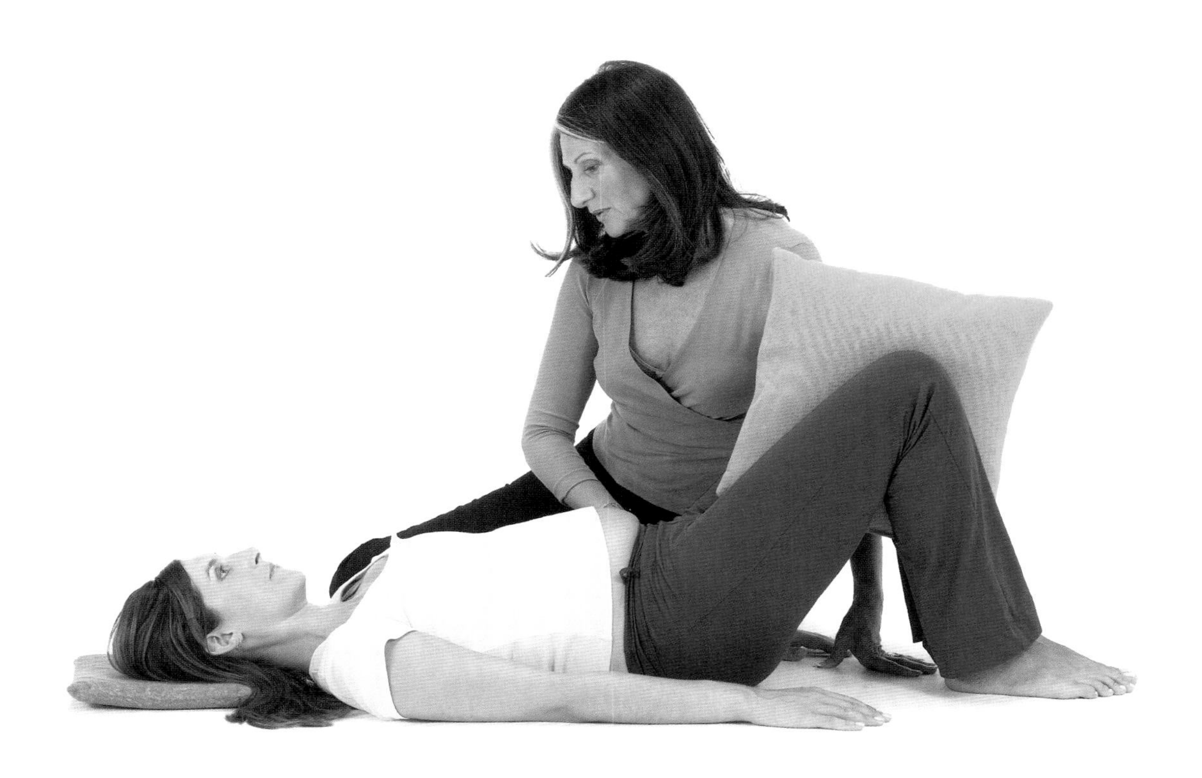

Walking on the Spot

A wonderful exercise for waking up the circulation in your legs, which helps prevent swelling. It's useful if you ever feel dizzy and cannot sit down, because it gets the deep calf pump working and your blood flowing.

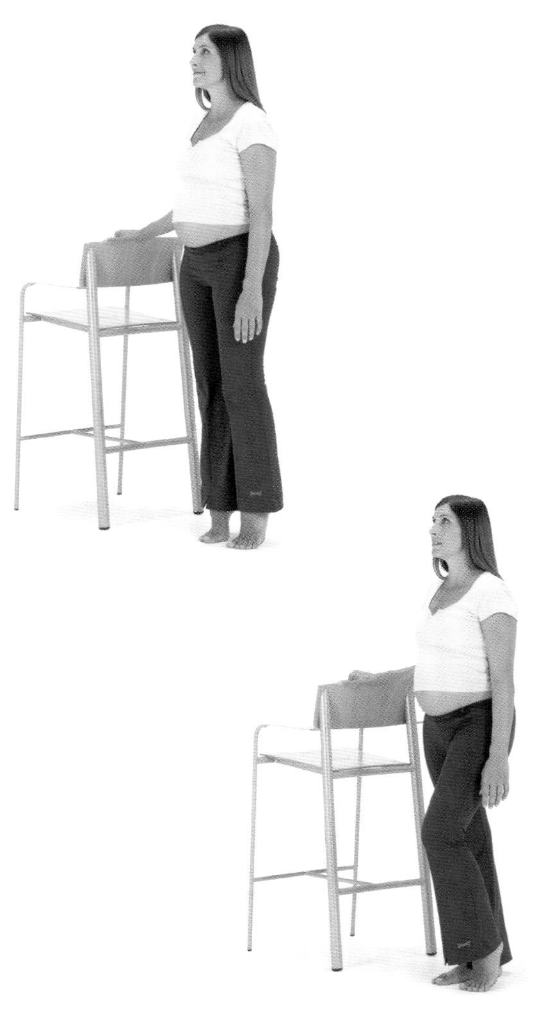

Aim

To warm up the legs, mobilizing the ankle joints, reaffirming good leg alignment and gently stretching the calves. It also gets the circulation going.

The key to doing this exercise well is to keep good body alignment throughout. You have three main body weights, your head, your ribcage and your pelvis. Try to keep them balanced centrally on top of each other. When you bend your knees they should bend directly over the second toes. You may have to check this occasionally during the exercise.

Starting Position

You may need to hold on to a wall or the back of a high chair. Stand correctly (page 16). Your feet are a little closer together than usual, just a few centimetres apart this time.

Action

1. Breathing normally, zip up and hollow and stay zipped and hollowed throughout. Come up on to the balls of both feet. Lower one heel down, staying on the ball of the other foot. The knee bends slightly (check it is bent directly over the centre of your foot). Change legs, transferring your weight. Do not wiggle your hips. Keep lengthening up, up, up and keep the waist long.
2. Continue walking on the spot for a couple of minutes.

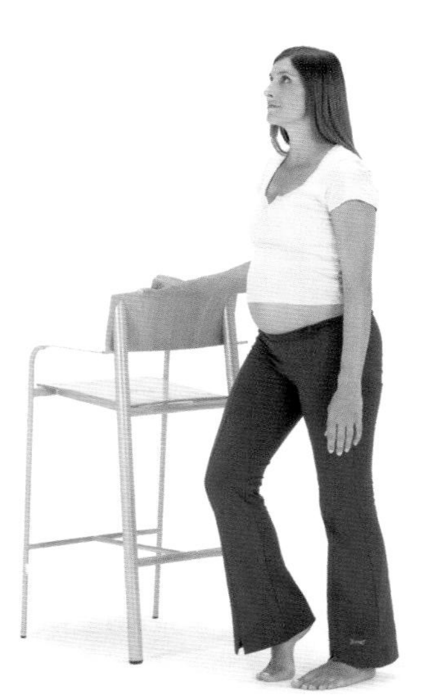

Watchpoints

- Try to keep your pelvis level, no wiggling.
- Try to use your zip up muscles to hold up your bump.
- Every so often check that your knees are bending straight over your second toes.
- Keep the action smooth and flowing.

The Corkscrew

This is nice to do if you are feeling as though you need a little more room in your abdomen!

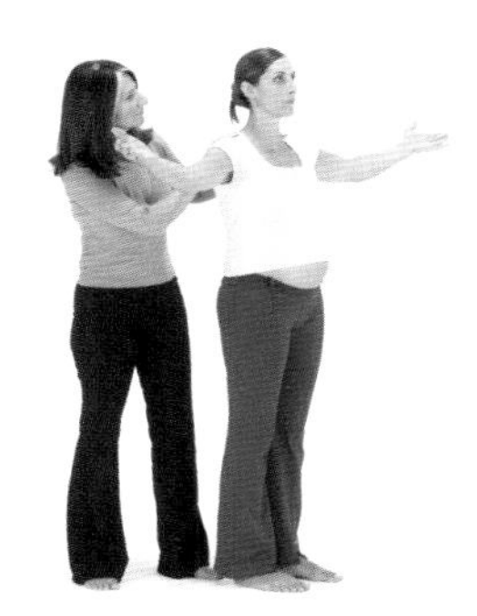

Aim

To learn the correct alignment and mechanics of the shoulders. To open the chest.

Why is it called the corkscrew? Imagine the type of corkscrew where as the arms are brought down the cork pops up – this is like your head coming up as your arms descend.

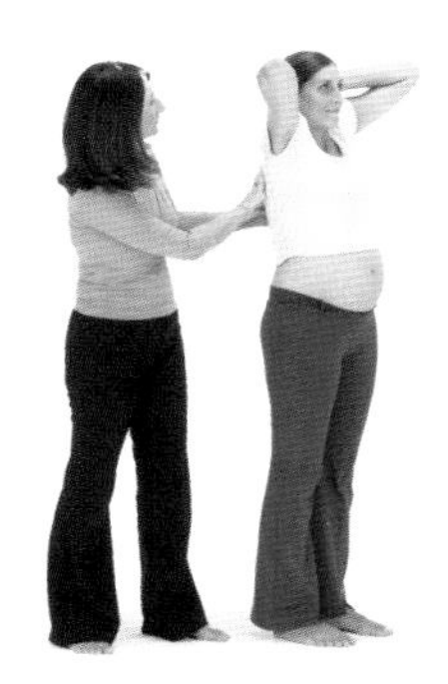

Starting Position

Stand correctly (page 16).

Action

1. Breathe in to prepare and lengthen up through the spine.
2. Breathe out, zip up and hollow and stay zipped and hollowed throughout. Allow your arms to float upwards. Keep the upper shoulders relaxed. Think of dropping the shoulder blades down into your back as the arms rise. Clasp your hands lightly behind your head.
3. Breathe in as you shrug your shoulders up to your ears.
4. Breathe out as you drop them down.
5. Breathe in as you move your elbows back a little. Your shoulder blades will come together slightly.
6. Breathe out as you release your hands and slowly bring them down by your sides, opening them wide and engaging the muscles beneath your shoulder blades. Allow the head, neck and spine to lengthen up as the arms come down. Think of a corkscrew.
7. Repeat up to 4 times. Do not do too many of these at once. It's better to come back and do a few more later.

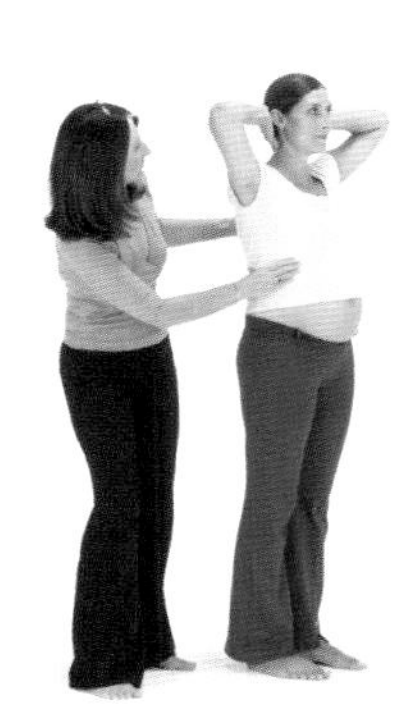

Watchpoints

- Remember not to arch the back as you bring your elbows back.
- As you bring the arms up, remember how the shoulder blades should move on the ribcage: they coil around. Try to keep the shoulder blades down for as long as possible by using the muscles in the back below them.
- Keep your arms in your peripheral vision at all times.

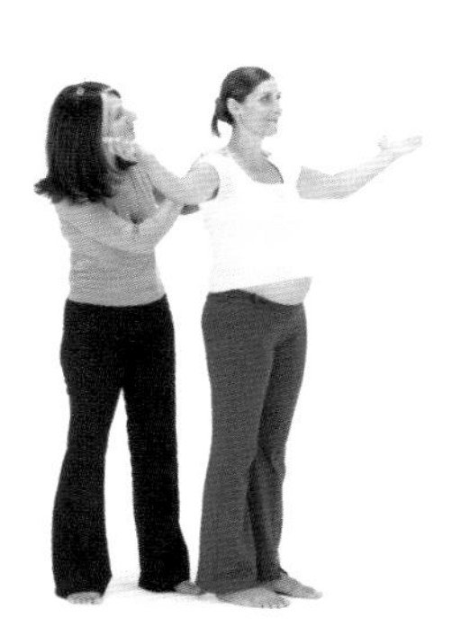

Bow and Arrow

A wonderful exercise that opens the upper body and teaches you to turn while lengthening. You should avoid big twisting movements, although you will naturally be turning around during your daily activities. Try to remember to lengthen up as you do so.

Aim
To learn to lengthen as you rotate the spine. Also to work the waist.

Equipment
A cushion and a towel.

Starting Position
Sit tall with your legs bent in front of you. You will probably prefer to have your knees a little apart to allow room for your bump. If you do, place a cushion between the knees and squeeze it gently throughout to help keep your legs and pelvis in line. Make sure you are sitting on your sitting bones. Put a rolled-up towel under your sitting bones if you wish. Hold your arms out in front of you, at shoulder height, palms facing down. Your shoulder blades are down into your back and your neck is released.

Action
1. Breathe in wide and full and lengthen through the spine.
2. Breathe out, zip up and hollow and stay zipped and hollowed throughout.
3. Breathe in and fold one hand in towards your chest. The elbow stays up in a line with the shoulder.
4. Still on the in-breath, follow the action through as you turn the upper body, unfolding the arm and straightening it out behind you. Your head follows the action but stays in a line with your spine. Your upper body is now open. Keep your knees together.
5. Breathe out and bring the arm back to the front in a wide circle.
6. Repeat 3 times to each side. You can help the rotation through the body by imagining that your straight arm is being pulled by a piece of string.

Watchpoints
- Keep lengthening up through the spine; don't allow the waist to sag.
- Keep your arms at shoulder height.
- Keep the shoulder blades down into your back.
- Keep the movements slow and flowing.

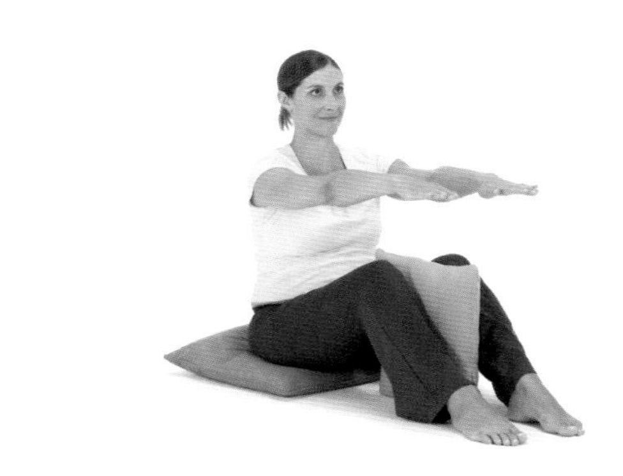

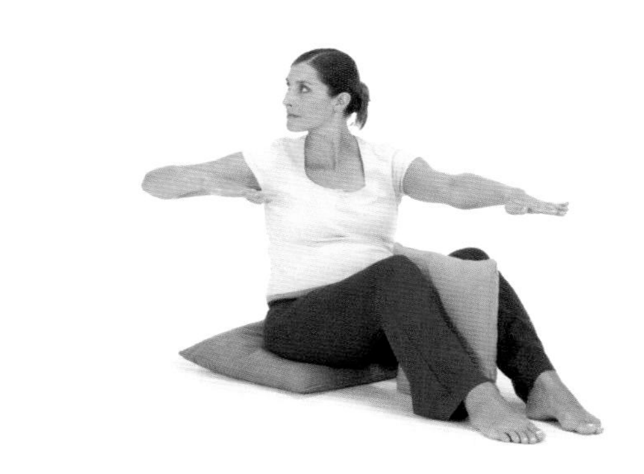

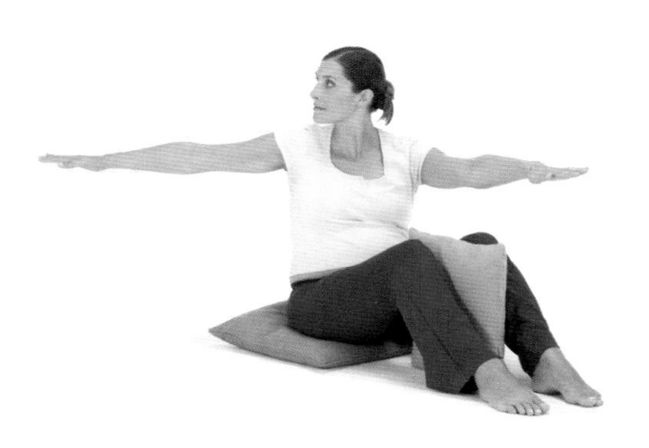

The Pillow Squeeze

Great for strengthening the inner thighs and opening the back.

Aim
To isolate and work the pelvic floor in conjunction with the deep abdominals, engaging the deep stabilizers. To strengthen the adductors. To learn the correct position of the pelvis. To 'open' the sacroiliac joints.

Equipment
A plump cushion.

Starting Position
Lie in the Relaxation Position (page 26) with your feet together, flat on the floor. Place a cushion between your knees. If your cushion is large, then you can have your feet a few centimetres apart, but line them up.

IMPORTANT NOTE

You will need to change position regularly every 3 minutes if you are in your last two trimesters.

Action

1. Breathe in wide and full to prepare.
2. Breathe out and zip up and hollow. Squeeze the cushion between your knees. Keep the pelvis in neutral and the tailbone down on the floor, lengthening away. Try not to grip around the hips. Continue to breathe normally, squeezing and working the pelvic floor and deep abdominals, for a count of up to 6. Then release.
3. Repeat 5 times.

Watchpoints

- Do not hold your breath; keep breathing.
- Keep your neck released and your jaw soft. You do not need to use your neck to work the pelvic floor!
- The most common mistake made doing this exercise is to lift the tailbone and tuck the pelvis. Think of keeping the length in the front of the pelvis, do not curl or shorten it. Another good way to check if you are tilting, is to place your hand under your waist. If you do the exercise wrong initially and tuck the pelvis, you will feel the pressure on your hand, as you push into the spine. Now try to do the exercise with no pressure on the hand – you have stayed in neutral.

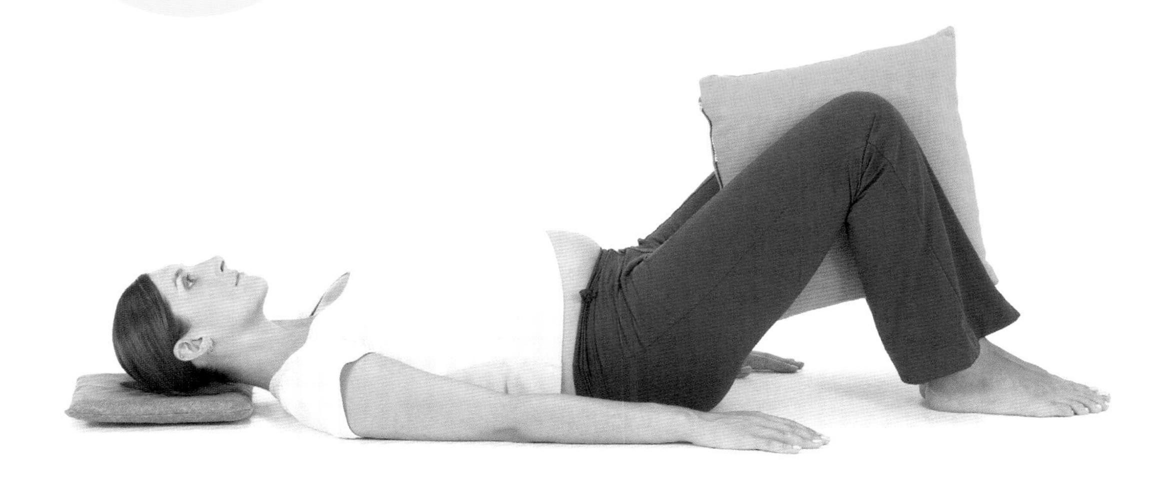

Monkey Bends

As your pregnancy progresses, you should start to include lots of squatting exercises. The action of squatting opens the pelvic outlet in readiness for the birth.

Aim

This subtle exercise opens the pelvis and also works on lengthening your spine and strengthening your postural muscles.

Starting Position

Stand well, feet hip-width apart and in parallel. Place your hands on the front of your thighs.

Action

1. Breathe in wide and lengthen through the top of your head.
2. Breathe out, zip up and hollow and stay zipped and hollowed throughout. Bend your knees directly over the centre of each foot, simultaneously, hingeing forward, pivoting from the hip joint. Slide your hands down your thighs. Keep your back long and in one piece with the head and neck. Think of the top of your head lengthening away from your tailbone.
3. Breathe in and lengthen back up to standing tall.
4. Repeat 5 times.

Watchpoints

- Keep your weight evenly distributed between both feet.
- Keep the back of the neck long and released.

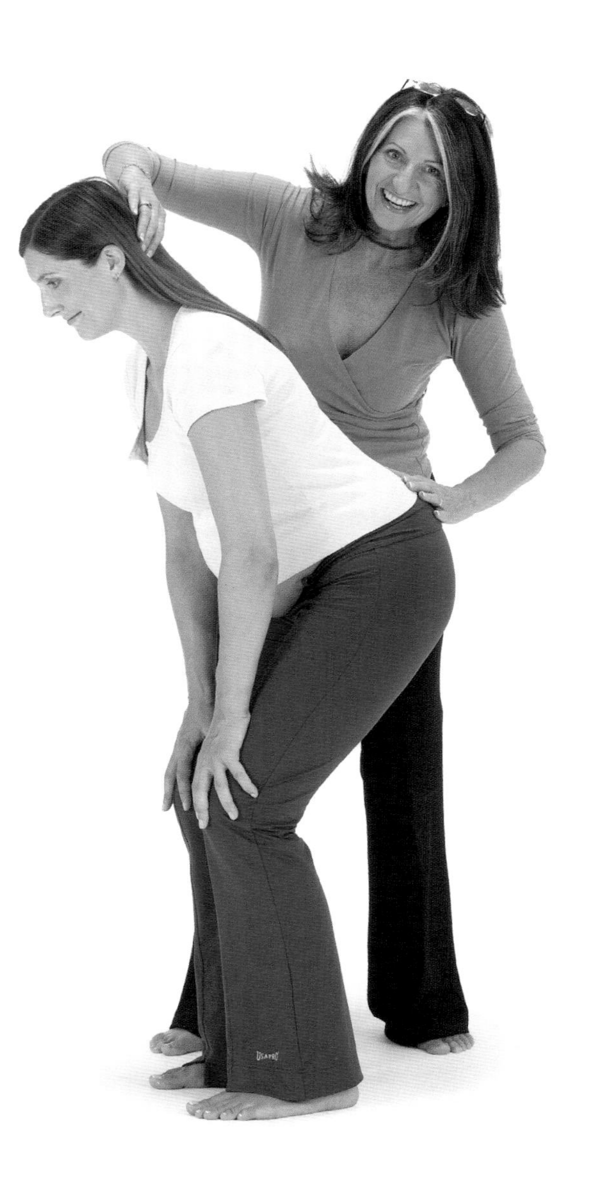

Monkey Bends with Arms

We have added an arm movement here, which is identical to Shoulder Reach (page 57). Try to keep your movements slow and flowing and co-ordinated.

Starting Position
Stand well, feet hip-width apart and in parallel. Have your arms down by your sides.

Action

1. Breathe in wide and lengthen through the top of your head.
2. Breathe out, zip up and hollow and stay zipped and hollowed throughout. Bend your knees directly over the centre of each foot, simultaneously hingeing forward, pivoting from the hip joint. At the same time, raise both arms out in front of you to shoulder height; keep the arms in an open 'C' shape, elbows softly bent.
3. Breathe in and lengthen back up to standing tall.
4. Repeat 5 times.

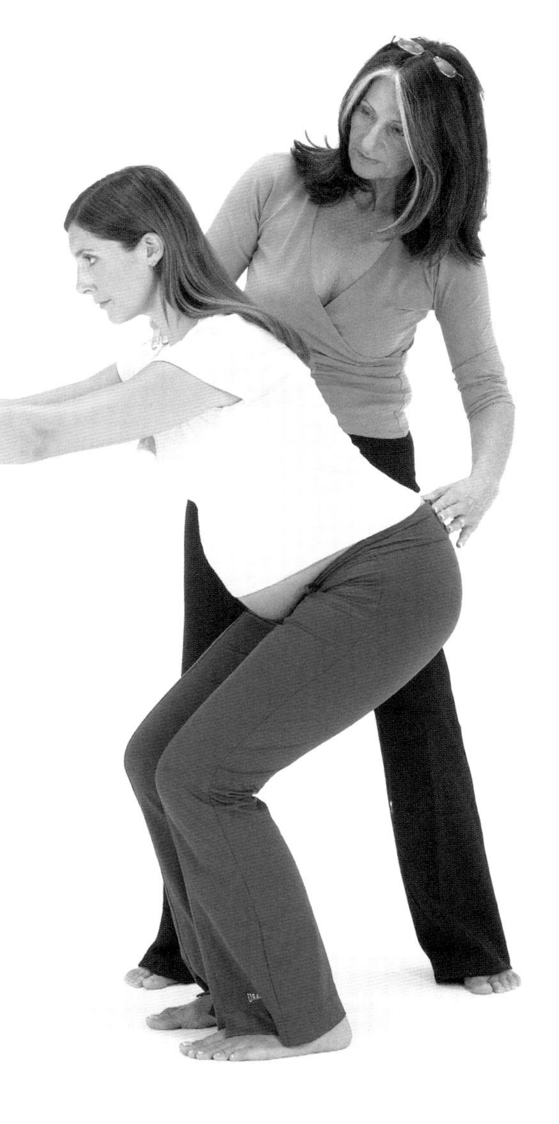

Watchpoints
As for Monkey Bends plus:

- Keep your back long and in one piece with the head and neck. Think of the top of your head lengthening away from your tailbone.
- Keep the shoulder blade connection – as the arms rise, they glide downwards.

Calf Stretch

There is a possibility that you will be suffering from leg cramps, particularly at night. This exercise helps relieve them.

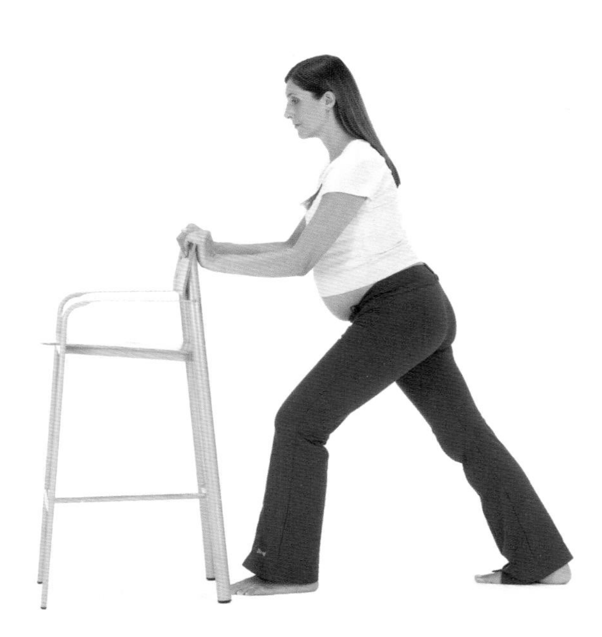

Starting Position and Action

1. Stand facing a wall or a tall stool. Place your hands and lower arms (with your elbows bent) against the wall. Put the toes of one foot against the base of the wall or stool bent in line with the ankle. The other leg should be behind the front one and should be straight, but not locked at the knee. The toes should be pointing forward with the heel down creating a stretch in the calf muscles.
2. Keep the weight spread evenly through the feet between the big toes, small toes and heels.
3. Repeat with the other leg.

Watchpoint

- Keep the breathing relaxed and even as you hold the stretch for about 20 seconds. Keep lengthening upwards. Keep zipping and hollowing.

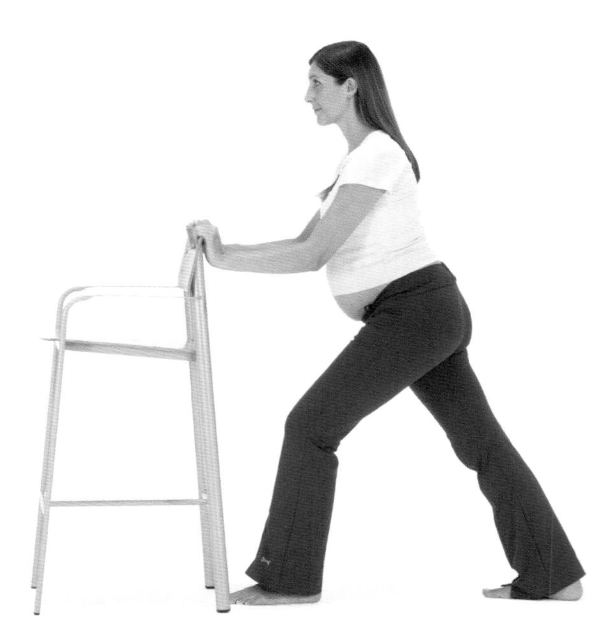

Chest Expansion

As your bump grows, it will become difficult for you to do back extensions lying on your front, but it is important that you include some form of back extension in your workout to compensate for any forward bending you have done either in your workout or in your daily activities. In this simple chest expansion exercise, make sure that you extend only the upper back and do not take the extension into your lumbar spine.

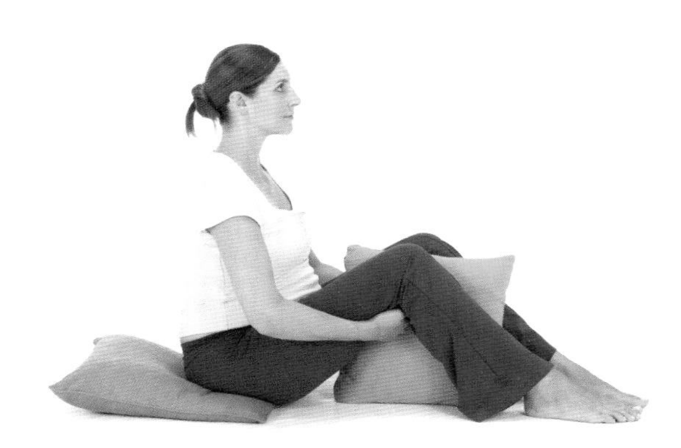

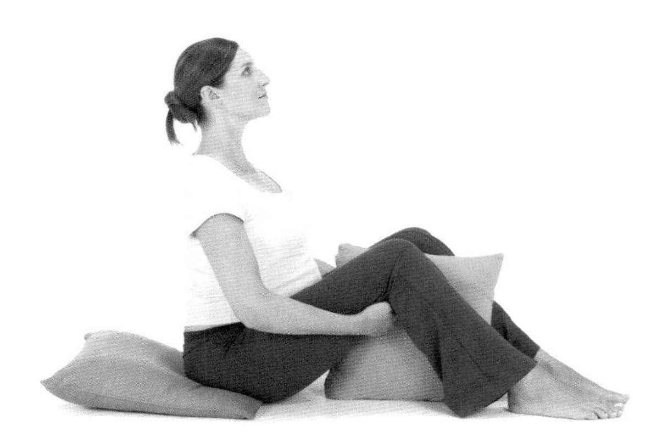

Equipment
A cushion, and a towel or a cushion.

Starting Position
Sit on the floor with a rolled-up towel or a cushion under your sitting bones. Your knees are bent and your feet are firmly planted on the floor, wider than hip-width apart (wherever they are comfortable). Put a cushion between your knees. Remember the triangle – base of the big toes, base of the small toes, centre of the heels. Hold your legs firmly behind the thighs, just above the back of the knees.

Action
1. Breathe in to prepare and lengthen up through the spine.
2. Breathe out and zip up and hollow. Imagine there is a cord attached to your breastbone, pulling it forward and up, opening the chest towards the ceiling. Your gaze can follow an arc and will stop where the wall meets the ceiling. Do not go back further. The neck stays long. Your ribcage stays down, integrated with your waist – think of your shoulder blades sliding down your back.
3. Breathe in and then, as you breathe out, slowly come to upright again, taking your gaze back down in an arc to where you started.
4. Repeat 5 times.

Watchpoints
- The feet stay planted into the floor.
- Move slowly and with control.
- Do not take the head back too far; it should move naturally with the movement of the spine.

NOTE

Please avoid this exercise if you have lumbar-sacral problems. Stop at any time if you feel dizzy.

Windows

Another lovely exercise for when you are feeling a little cramped!

Aim
To open the upper body and teach good mechanics. It also promotes flexibility and mobility around the shoulder joint.

Equipment
A broomstick or a scarf.

Starting Position
Lie in the Relaxation Position (page 26). Raise your arms directly above your shoulders, with the palms facing away from you. Your shoulder blades remain down into your back, your upper body relaxed and open.

Action
1. Breathe in wide and full to prepare.
2. Breathe out, zip up and hollow and stay zipped and hollowed throughout. Bring your elbows down towards the floor, keeping your arms bent. Your upper arms are in a line with the shoulders to each side.
3. Breathe in and very slowly rotate your arms backwards; the backs of your hands will come down towards the floor. Under no circumstances force the arms back. Stop where they are comfortable. Feel your shoulder blades connecting down into your back as you make this movement.
4. Breathe out as you slowly straighten the arms along the floor (or just off the floor if this is more comfortable), keeping them wide. Don't lock the elbows. Keep the action smooth and flowing, but don't forget the shoulder blade connection down in your back.
5. Breathe in as you raise the arms back to the Starting Position.
6. Repeat 5 times.

Watchpoints
- Make your movements smooth, controlled and without strain.
- Shoulder blades down at all times.
- Keep your ribcage and your breastbone soft.

IMPORTANT NOTE

You will need to change position regularly every 3 minutes if you are in your last two trimesters

NOTE

Please take advice if you have a shoulder injury.

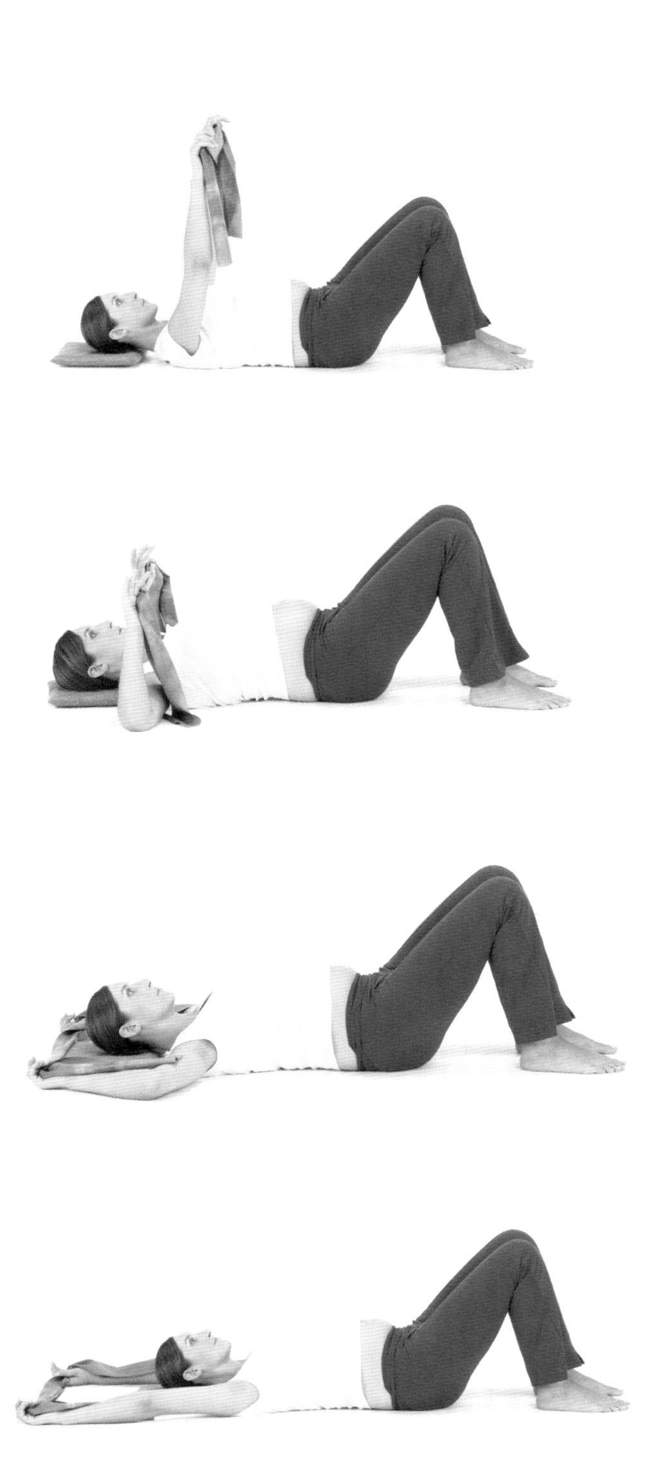

Side-lying Circles

Lying on your side will feel really good as you get bigger. The beauty of this exercise is that you are making very small movements, yet isolating the buttocks very precisely.

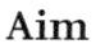

Aim
To work the buttocks or thighs.

Equipment
A cushion or two.

Starting Position
Lie on your right side in a straight line. Place a cushion under your bump if you wish. Line up your joints, shoulder over shoulder, hip over hip. You can either stretch out your lower arm and rest your head on it, or prop your head up on your hand with the elbow bent. Bring both legs a little in front of you. This gives you greater stability.

Action
1. Breathe in and lengthen through the body.
2. Breathe out, zip up and hollow and stay zipped and hollowed throughout. Slowly lift your right leg and bring it back in a line with your body and to hip height – about 15 centimetres (6 inches) off the floor.
3. You can now either leave the leg in parallel or turn it out from the hip.
4. Breathing normally, draw 5 small circles in the air (about the size of a grapefruit), change direction and draw 5 the other way.
5. Return the upper leg to the lower leg. Turn over and repeat on the other side. You should feel this in your buttock.

Watchpoints
- Keep lengthening through the body; do not allow your waist (or what is left of it!) to sink into the floor.
- Keep the circles small and neat.
- Keep the movements free; the hip should be open.
- Keep good alignment through the body; the shoulders stay in line balanced on top of each other, shoulder blades down into the back, neck released.
- Keep zipping.

Sliding Down the Wall

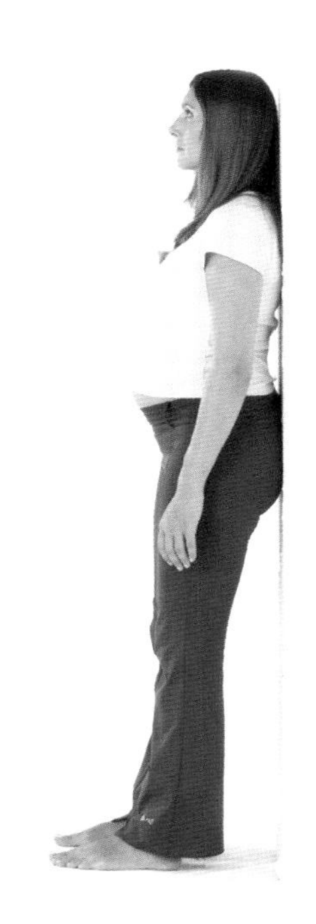

This exercise has many benefits: it works the thighs, stretches the calves and teaches good postural alignment. It is also a squatting action, which opens the pelvic outlet. We have given you two variations. If possible, try to decide whether your low back is over-arched or too flat – variation one is for the flat-backed pregnancy, variation two benefits mothers to be who have too much of a hollow in the low back.

Aim
To learn how to lengthen the base of the spine, achieving the correct angle of the pelvis to the spine. To work the thigh muscles and stretch the calf muscle.

For Flat Backs: Starting Position
Stand, with your back to the wall, and your feet about 15 centimetres (6 inches) away from it. Your feet are hip-width apart and parallel. Lean back into the wall. Don't try to force your head back on the wall, just stand comfortably. Before you begin, take note as to which parts of your back are touching the wall.

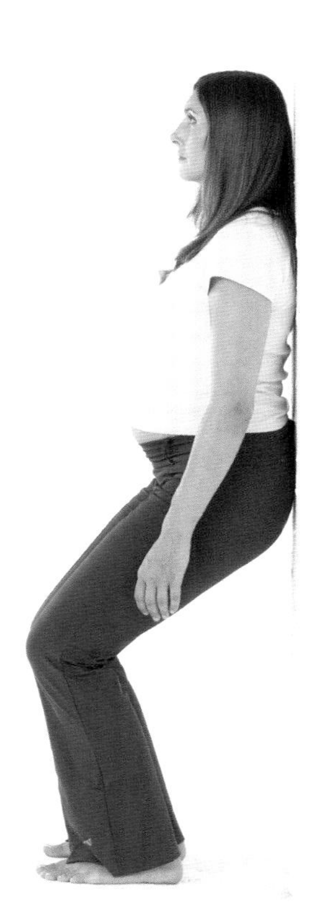

Action
1. Breathe in wide and full to prepare, lengthening through the spine.
2. Breathe out and zip up and hollow. Bend your knees and slide about 30 centimetres (12 inches) down the wall until your thighs are almost parallel with the floor – don't go any lower than this! Keep your feet flat on the floor (your heels will want to come up – don't let them). Don't allow your tailbone to lift off the wall, rather keep it lengthening away from you. Stay neutral; there should be a gentle stretch in your lumbar spine.
3. Breathe in as you slide back up, still zipping and trying to keep the base of the spine lengthened.
4. Repeat 5 times.

For Over-arched Backs: Starting Position
As for version one.

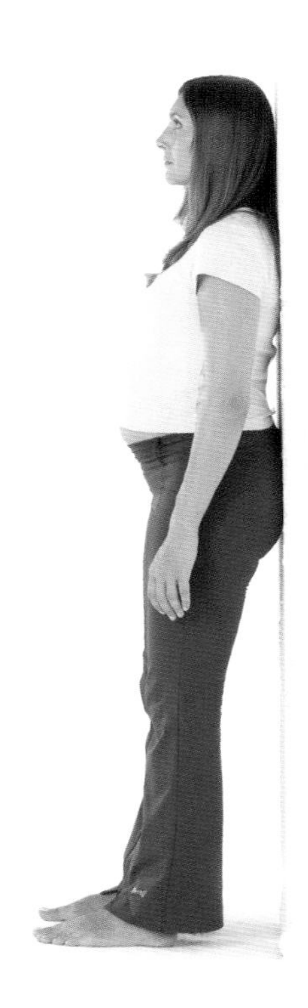

Action

1. Breathe in wide and full to prepare, lengthening through the spine.
2. Breathe out and zip up and hollow. Bend your knees and slide about 30 centimetres (12 inches) down the wall until your thighs are almost parallel with the floor – don't go any lower than this! As you slide down, gently press your low back into the wall, lengthening the base of the spine. Your tailbone should still stay on the wall but more of your low back should come into contact with the wall.
3. Breathe in as you slide back up, still zipping and trying to keep the base of the spine lengthened.
4. Repeat 5 times.

As you leave the wall, stand upright for a moment imagining that the wall is still there.

Watchpoints

- Watch that you don't slide down too far – you may not be able to get back up! Never take your bottom below knee level.
- Check that your knees are passing directly over your feet and not inside them. Your feet must stay parallel; don't let them roll inwards.
- Keep your heels on the floor; they will want to come up – don't let them.

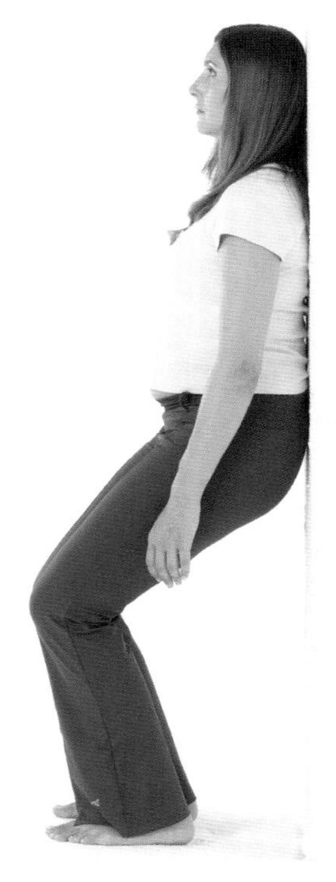

Arm Openings

A wonderful feel-good exercise. Everyone's favourite.

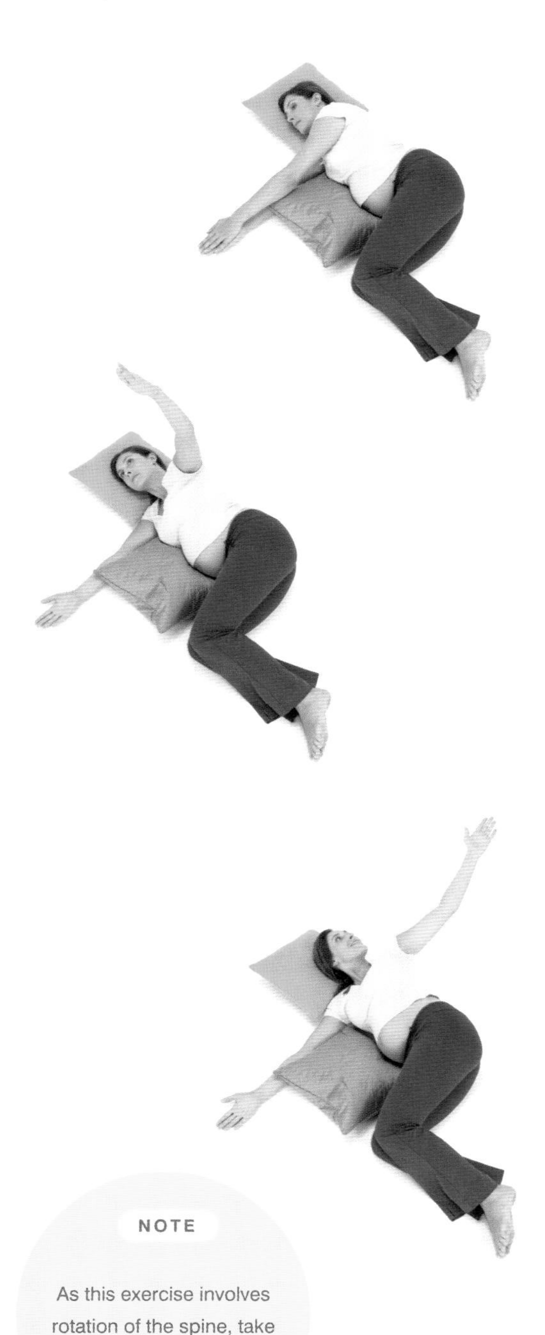

Aim

To open the upper body and stretch the pectoral muscles, while stabilizing the shoulder blades. To achieve a sense of 'openness' while stabilizing and centring. To gently and safely rotate the spine.

Equipment

Bedroom pillows or large cushions. You may need three.

Starting Position

Lie on your side with your head on a pillow and your knees bent at a right angle to your body. Your back should be in a straight line, but with its natural curves. Stack your bones up on top of each other, feet, ankles, knees, hips and shoulders. Place one pillow between your knees, but try to keep them in line. Put another pillow under your bump (optional) and the last one under your head. Your arms are extended in front of you, palms together, at shoulder height.

Action

1. Breathe in to prepare and lengthen through the spine.
2. Breathe out, and zip up and hollow.
3. Breathe in as you slowly lift the upper arm, keeping the elbow soft, and the shoulder blade down into the back. Keep your eyes on your hand so that the head follows the arm movement. You are aiming to touch the floor behind you, but do not force it. Try to keep your knees together and your pelvis still. Stay zipped and hollowed.
4. Breathe out as you bring the arm back in an arc to rest on the other hand again.
5. Repeat 5 times, then curl up on the other side and start again.

Watchpoints

- Keep hollowing throughout.
- Keep your waist long; don't let it to sink into the floor.
- Don't forget to allow your head to roll naturally with the movement. Make sure that it is supported by the pillow.
- Keep the gap between your ears and your shoulders by engaging the muscles below the shoulder blades.
- Stay completely aware of your arm and hand as it displaces the air moving through space.

NOTE

As this exercise involves rotation of the spine, take advice if you have a disc-related injury.

Second Trimester Workouts

There are 5 balanced workouts set out below. Each lasts approximately 20–30 minutes, and you should try to do all 5 workouts once each week.

The exercises are mainly drawn from this chapter but we have also added a few from earlier and later chapters which will make the workouts more varied. You can of course add any exercise from later in the book if you wish.

The workouts are designed so that you change position frequently. Everyone works at a different pace so you may need to cut the number of repetitions that you do if you have spent more than 3 minutes lying on your back.

NOTE

If you are finding it difficult to get down on and up from the floor see page 144.

Workout One

Sliding Down the Wall 135
Walking on the Spot 124
The Corkscrew 125
Baby Spine Curls with Pillow Squeeze 123
Bow and Arrow 126
Windows 132
Side-lying Circles 134
Pelvic Stability: Knee Folds and Knee Drops 55
Chest Expansion 131
Shoulder Drops 66
The Pelvic Elevator (sitting) 49
Arm Circles (With Weights) 104
Calf Stretch 130
The Pillow Squeeze 127

Workout Two

Demi Pliés in Turn Out 100
The Dumb Waiter 101
Single Leg Circles 102
Threading a Needle 110
The Rest Position 93
Baby Spine Curls with Pillow Squeeze 123
The Oyster 149
Hip Flexor Stretch 72
The Pelvic Elevator (sitting) 46
/ Emergency Stop 71
The Full Starfish 65
Chest Expansion 131
Arm Openings 137
Monkey Bends 129
Roll Downs Against the Wall 84

Workout Three

Walking on the Spot 124
Monkey Bends with Arms 129
Sitting Side Reach 86
Hip Rolls (Level One only) 81
Abductor and Adductor Lifts (no weights)
87 and 89
Windows 132
The Pelvic Elevator (sitting) 49
Bow and Arrow 126
Shoulder Drops 66
Chest Expansion 131
The Cat 155
Arm Circles (with weights) 104
The Rest Position 93
The Pillow Squeeze 127

Workout Four

Sliding Down the Wall 135
Floating Arms 59
Back Press 158
Sitting Tarzan 157
Arm Openings 137
The Pillow Squeeze 127
Side-lying Circles 134
Baby Spine Curls with Pillow Squeeze 123
The Pelvic Elevator (sitting) 49 / Emergency Stop 71
Hip Rolls (Level One only) 81
Chest Expansion 131
Hip Flexor Stretch 72
Calf Stretch 130
The Dumb Waiter 101
Demi Pliés in Turn Out 100

Workout Five

The Full Starfish 65
The Oyster 149
Baby Spine Curls with PIllow Squeeze 123
Arm Openings 137
Ankle Circles 112
Chest Expansion 131
Sliding Down the Wall 135
The Corkscrew 125
Arm Circles (With Weights) 104
Sitting Side Reach 86
Pelvic Elevator (sitting) 49
Pelvic Stability: Knee Folds and Knee Drops 55
Abductor and Adductor Lifts (no weights)
87 and 89
The Pillow Squeeze 127

9 The Third Trimester (27–34 weeks)

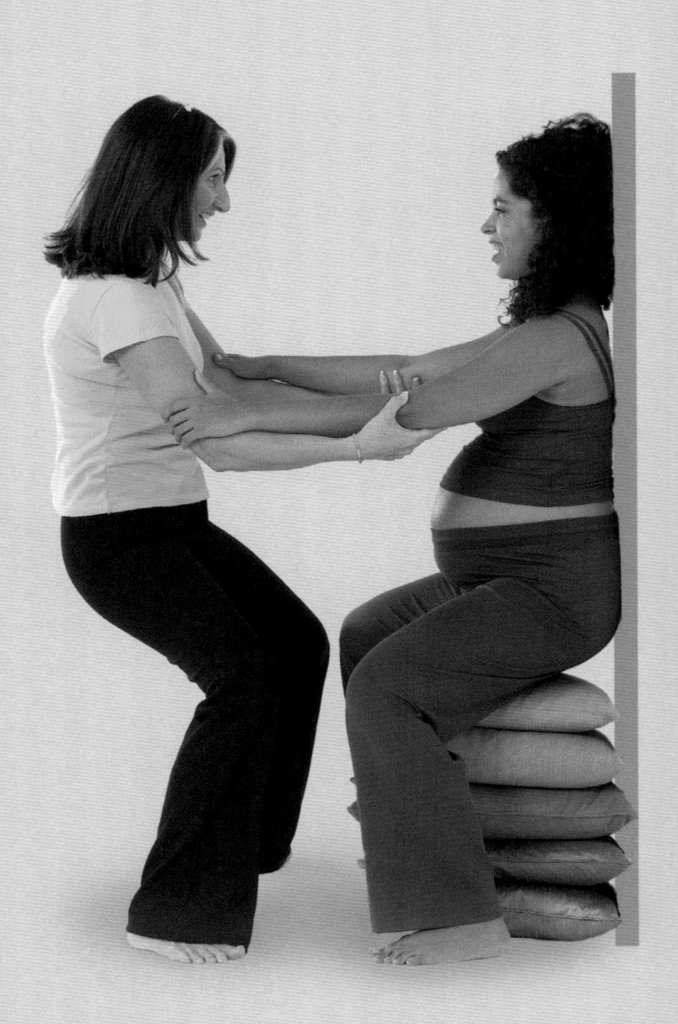

What's Happening to Your Body?

The last trimester can be the most uncomfortable for the mother to be because by the time you reach full term, the uterus is right up under the ribs and is very large! A pre-pregnant size of 5 to 10 centimetres (2 to 4 inches) has now increased to 25 to 36 centimetres (10 to 14 inches). It has increased 5 to 6 times in size and 20 times in weight!

A total weight gain of up to 15 kilos (33 pounds) is considered acceptable, but is at the top of the scale. By the birth, the baby will be 33 to 39 centimetres (12 to 15 inches) long and will weigh approximately 3 kilos (7 pounds). A range of beween 2.2 to 4.5 kilos (5 to10 pounds) is considered normal. In fact, the baby is now so big that he or she has less room to move in – so you will probably feel less movement but when you do, it will feel more like squirming than kicking!

As you become heavier and more restricted in your movements, it is even more important for you to practise Pilates. You may not feel as graceful as before, but there are enormous benefits to be had from exercising right up to the end, as long as you are feeling well, are pain free and are not displaying any of the contraindications listed on pages 22 and 23.

You will continue to be prone to a variety of conditions related to the increase in blood volume, the size of the uterus, fluid retention, and the hormonal effects on muscle tissue and ligaments, as discussed in the opening chapters.

The advice given for the second trimester will continue to apply through this trimester:

- Keep your workouts short to avoid fatigue.
- Avoid doing too many repetitions.
- Change position slowly and frequently, taking your time to move from one exercise to the next, rolling on to your left side when coming up, see page 144.
- Don't do too many standing exercises in a row.
- Watch the clock to make sure you do not spend longer than 3 minutes on your back.

We have given you a few side-lying exercises which are very useful at this stage. A cushion under your bump helps support you.

Curl-up exercises are still forbidden, but remember that if you have done Pilates throughout your pregnancy you will have a natural girdle of strength so keep zipping up and hollowing or zipping and lifting your bump!

You must ensure you get plenty of rest. Your blood pressure will be very closely monitored by your antenatal clinic, because it can rise during this period. High blood pressure is a symptom of pre-eclampsia, which affects 5–10 per cent of pregnant women and, if left unchecked, it can lead to eclampsia – a very serious condition for both mother and baby (see page 22). To help keep your stress levels low, make sure your workouts include plenty of relaxation exercises such as Shoulder Drops (page 66) and Neck Rolls and Chin Tucks (page 62). A few gentle exercises before you go to bed may still your mind and help you sleep. You are going to need lots of 'me' time and time to put your feet up, but you must also stay active and fit in preparation for the hard work of labour and motherhood!

From about your twentieth week, your uterus has been rehearsing for the birth itself with practice contractions, known as Braxton Hicks. You may not have noticed these before, but as you reach the end of this trimester, the contractions can become strong enough to be uncomfortable. Many mothers to be have dashed off to hospital thinking they were in labour, so powerful were their Braxton Hicks! You are not going to hurt the baby or yourself by doing a Pilates session when you are having Braxton Hicks, but you may find it difficult to zip up and hollow while the uterus tightens and flexes its muscles. Occasionally, zipping up and hollowing can set the Braxton Hicks off. If this is the case, then you will have to stop the session and try again later.

The indigestion, flatulence and heartburn that you probably started to suffer in the last trimester tend to get worse in this third trimester. You can blame the hormones progesterone and relaxin, which are produced in large quantities during pregnancy. They are responsible for relaxing the muscle tissue throughout the body and this, unfortunately, also includes the gastrointestinal tract. As a result, your food passes much more slowly through your digestive system, making you prone to indigestion and flatulence. On the plus side, it means that more nutrients are absorbed. Heartburn can be a real nuisance. It is caused in pregnancy by the relaxation of the ring of muscle that separates the oesophagus from the stomach. Food and digestive juices can thus back up. Bear this in mind when deciding when to do your sessions. Remember, too, that good posture will help your digestion. You may find that exercises such as the Corkscrew (page 125) and Pole Raises (page 152) will help to relieve the pressure on your stomach.

You will also experience respiratory changes mainly due to fluid retention and to the simple fact that the uterus is pushing up on the diaphragm and causing the lower ribs to lift and flare and you may find yourself short of breath. This does not mean however that either you or the baby will be short of oxygen! The changes actually allow you to take in more oxygen. You may feel as though you need to breathe more deeply but can't. The lateral thoracic breathing that you have been practising in Pilates will help you here, but be kind to yourself – sometimes your breath will have to be more shallow. Good posture will help your breathing. Slouching will only close the ribcage down and restrict your breathing, so stand and sit tall. You may find you have to alter the breathing from the directions given in the exercises. This is fine. The main thing to remember is not to over breathe or you may make yourself dizzy, and never ever hold your breath while exercising.

The increased weight of the uterus will put a further strain on the spine. As oestrogen levels rise, your joints will continue to be more mobile than normal so good alignment and lots of stability exercises are now crucial. However, you may in fact become more stable in the lumbar pelvic area. This is because the sheer weight and size of the uterus, bolted as it is on to your front, acts a little like a full-blown sail would to a sailing boat, stabilizing you.

If this is your first child, then about 2 to 4 weeks before the birth, the baby's head may engage. This is known as the lightening, and occurs when the presenting part of the baby (hopefully the head!) drops into the upper bony part of the pelvis in readiness for the birth. It doesn't always happen before labour, and with second and subsequent pregnancies it usually happens during labour itself rather than before. As the baby's head engages there is less pressure on the ribcage – making breathing easier. The bad news is that there is now more pressure on the pelvic floor which must withstand the weight of the uterus. It can drop as much as 2.5 centimetres (1 inch). As we mentioned in the opening chapter, the pelvic floor lies at the bottom of the abdomino-pelvic cavity. Your pelvic floor exercises are now vital. As Sheila Kitzinger writes in her book *The New Pregnancy and Childbirth*, your baby will now be using your pelvic floor as a trampoline! Remember the image of a cardboard box full of heavy bottles? How would you carry it? From the sides only? No! You would support it from underneath!!!! So, lots of pelvic floor exercises please. The Emergency Stop (page 71) will help prevent accidents when you cough or sneeze.

Now is the time to start thinking about the birth itself, so you will also need to learn how to release those pelvic floor muscles. You have to learn how to let go. Exercises such as the Flower (page 160) and taking the lift down to the basement in the Pelvic Floor Release (page 159) will help give you the right sensation. They may also help prevent stress incontinence.

One of our main aims in this final trimester is to create space for the baby to move around in. More than ever you need to focus on lengthening, widening and opening the body. Although your abdominals are strong, over the last few months you have been working on the wrap-around abdominals, transversus abdominis, rather than the six-pack muscles, rectus abdominis, thus allowing plenty of room for your baby to grow. Remember too that transversus is your pushing muscle when you are in labour.

Four-point kneeling is a position which (unless you suffer from carpal tunnel syndrome) should feel wonderful because it takes the weight of the baby off the spine and pubic bone. The Cat (page 155) is a lovely way to mobilize your spine, but it will be harder to do in pregnancy than before because you have to lift the bump (your very own built-in training weight!). Another good way to prepare for the birth is to practise squatting. This is a favourite birth position because it helps open up the pelvic outlet. Monkey Bends (page 128) and Sliding Down the Wall (page 135) are also helpful and we have given you another squatting exercise for the last few weeks.

There is one thing that should be mentioned here, even though the chances of it happening are very, very rare. Sometimes, with certain movements, air is drawn into the vagina. Normally this is no problem (except, perhaps, for the embarrassing noise it can make!) but in a pregnant woman there is a slight risk of an air embolism occurring as the pressure change causes air to be sucked into the vagina and the uterus, where it can enter the circulatory system through an open placenta wound. There is particular danger if there is any bleeding or other symptoms of early placental displacement. There is more risk of this in the six weeks after the birth. Basically, you should avoid movements or positions which force air into the vagina, e.g. coming up from Rest Position where the buttocks may be elevated, drawing the knee to the chest in four-point kneeling, or any position, coming down from a shoulder stand in yoga, for example, where the buttocks are elevated and the uterus moves upwards. We have deliberately avoided such movements in the third trimester programme but if you are including other fitness techniques in your schedule, you must be aware of the potential dangers of such movements.

Getting on to and up from the Floor in the Third Trimester and up to Six Weeks After the Birth

- Slowly lower yourself on to one knee.
- Then come on to both knees.
- Place both hands on the floor in front of you and carefully move so you sit to one side.
- Now, zip up and hollow and bring your legs in front of you. Very slowly and, with control, zipping all the time, lower yourself back using your elbows to support you.
- To come back up, roll on to your side, keeping your knees bent.
- Use your hands to push yourself into a side-sitting position.
- Then come on to all fours.
- Bring one knee in front.
- With your hand on your knee, push yourself into a standing position.

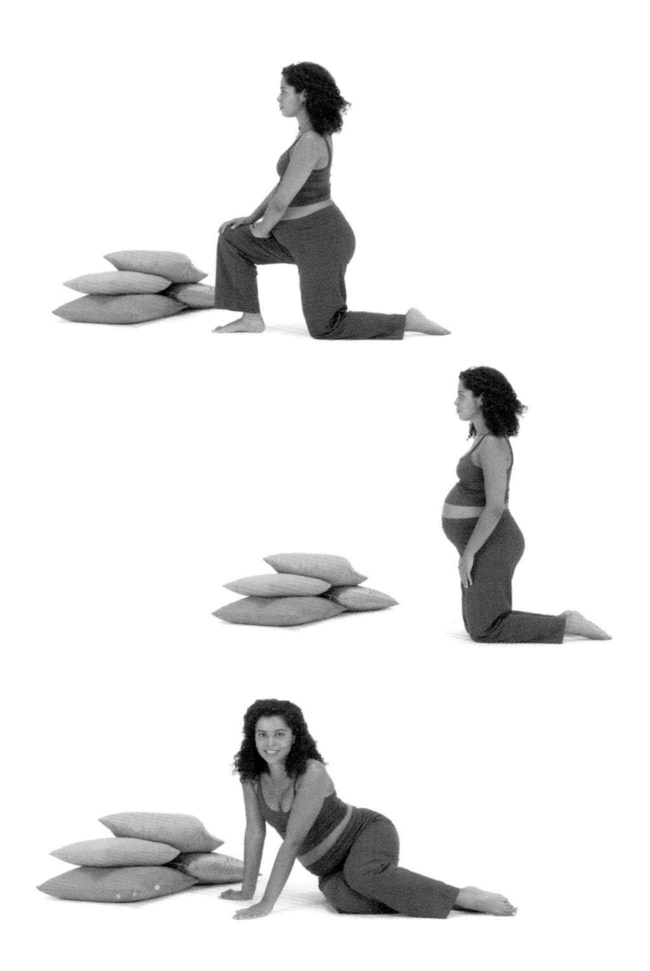

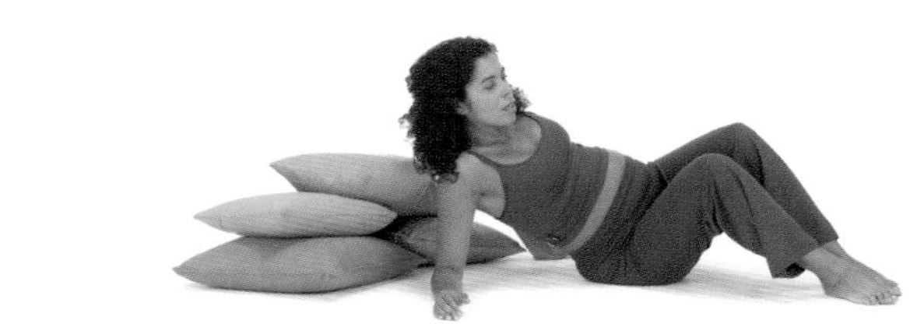

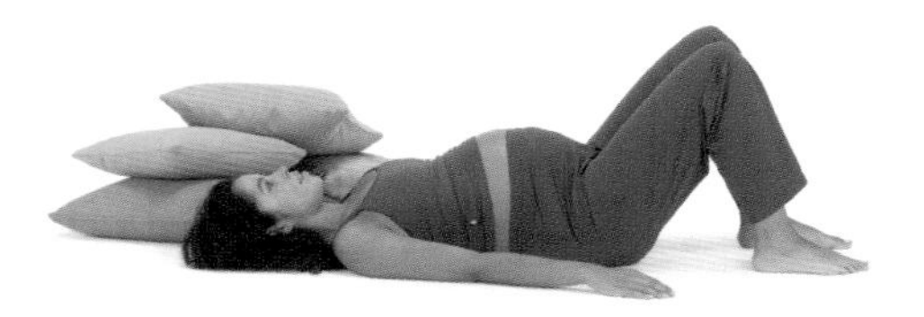

Guidelines for Exercising in the Third Trimester

Continue to follow all the advice given on page 121 for the second trimester. They are recapitulated here to remind you.

I did Pilates all though my pregnancy confident that I never exceeded what I should be doing safely. I didn't suffer a bit of backache. And, more importantly, I was still in my Earl jeans until the last couple of months!'

– Harriet Green

- Keep sessions a manageable length so you do not tire.
- Take extra care as you will be a little clumsy and your balance will be affected.
- Be careful when moving from one position to the next – allow extra time. If coming up from lying, roll on to your side and then wait a moment and rise slowly, see opposite.
- Do fewer repetitions of exercises.
- Plan your sessions to take into account meal times and any indigestion you may suffer. If indigestion is bad, try exercises that raise the arms, but do not over reach.
- Do not spend longer than 3 minutes lying on your back; change positions frequently.
- If you feel at all dizzy then lie on your left side – this is also an ideal position for resting.
- Try to include some back extensions such as Chest Expansion (page 131) at each workout. But take care not to allow the low back to over hollow or extend.
- Continue with the zip up and hollow action, even though there is not much in the way of a hollow. Zip and lift.
- Take a moment to relax between exercises so that your abdominals can have a break.
- Always include exercises for scapular stability, such as the Corkscrew (page 125) and Windows (page 132), to prevent poor posture and, in particular, to prevent you becoming round shouldered and to help support the added weight of the breasts.
- Identify how your posture is changing/has changed and choose your exercises accordingly.

- Avoid any exercise which involves curling up from the mat (flexion). Therefore, no Curl Ups, Single Leg Stretches, Hundreds, etc.

- Include exercises which elevate the legs and work the calf pump to help improve circulation, do Ankle Circles for example on page 112, but do not spend more than 3 minutes in this position.

- Include calf stretches to help prevent leg cramps.

- Because of instability around the pelvis, you should continue to avoid exercises with a wide range of movement and/or long levers. Do not use leg weights. Arm weights are fine.

- Hamstring and adductor stretches should be used with caution. Overstretching these muscle groups can increase pelvic instability or hypermobility.

- Avoid exercises which put any pressure on the pubis symphysis. This is liable to separate with the increased laxity of the ligaments, e.g. Sitting Wide Leg Stretch.

- Avoid holding positions or stretches for long periods of time.

- Try not to do too many standing positions in a row.

- Take care with balancing or weight-bearing exercises on one leg. This may promote sacroiliac or pubis symphysis discomfort.

- You might like to use a wedge or a rolled-up towel under the sitting bones in sitting exercises.

- Empty your bladder before a workout to save you having to interrupt the session and to avoid mishaps.

- Change the timing of the breathing if you need to if, for example, you are short of breath. Never hold your breath.

- Do lots of pelvic floor exercises, but they should now include release work, e.g. the Flower (page 160) or the Pelvic Elevator (page 70) going down to the basement, to prepare for the birth.

- Four-point kneeling exercises will feel wonderful because they take the weight of the baby off the spine and pubic bone, but take care if you have carpal tunnel syndrome; use a rolled-up towel.

- Include Pilates-style squats, because they are good for circulation and in preparation for the birth.

- Get the calf pump working to help circulation – with Walking on the Spot (page 124), Tennis Ball Rises (page 154), Sliding Down the Wall (page 135).

- If Braxton Hicks contractions are interfering with your workout, stop and try again later. They may be uncomfortable and it is hard to exercise through them, but they are perfectly normal. Rarely, abdominal hollowing may set them off!

IMPORTANT NOTE

Don't forget to ask your midwife at each antenatal check up, 'Is it OK for me to continue with Pilates?'

Recommended Exercises for the Third Trimester

Arm Circles Against the Wall

You can use very light weights for this exercise, which makes it good for toning the arms.

Aim

To mobilize the shoulder girdle and to improve scapular stabilizing skills.

Try to move your hands along the wall while keeping the body well aligned, but work within your comfort range. It is better to keep the ribcage down and not arch the back than force the arms back.

Equipment

Light weights of 0.5 kilo (1 pound) each weight (optional).

Starting Position

Stand comfortably with your back against the wall and your feet about 15 centimetres (6 inches) away from it. Your feet are hip-width apart and parallel. Check that your pelvis is in neutral and your knees are soft. Use the wall to help keep good alignment throughout the body.

Action

1. Breathe in wide and full to prepare.
2. Breathe out, zip up and hollow and stay zipped and hollowed throughout. Reach your arms out in front of you, with your palms down, and take them above your head.
3. Lengthen through your fingers and keep your shoulder blades drawing down into your back.
4. As you breathe in, reach your arms out to the sides, with the palms facing forwards, and lengthen them down to the sides of your body.
5. Repeat 6 times. Then, reverse the circle, exhaling as the arms lift up, and inhaling as the arms lower down.

Watchpoints

- Maintain neutral pelvis and neutral spine throughout and do not allow the upper back to arch away from the wall.
- Do not allow the ribs to flare. Move with the breath.
- Keep the shoulder blades wide and down the back, but do allow for mobility. No gripping!
- Keep the neck long and released.
- Watch the alignment of the hands and wrists!
- Keep the elbows soft.

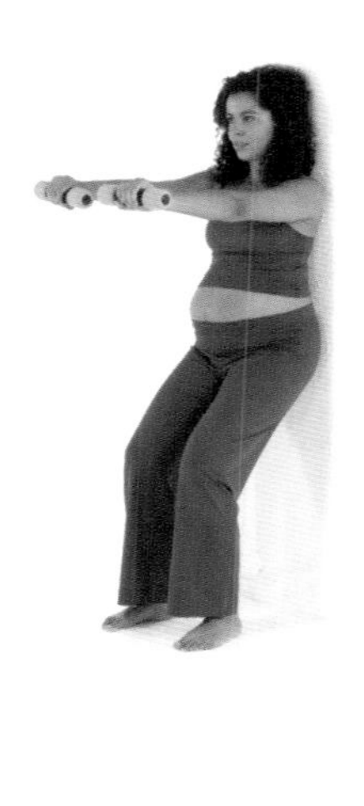
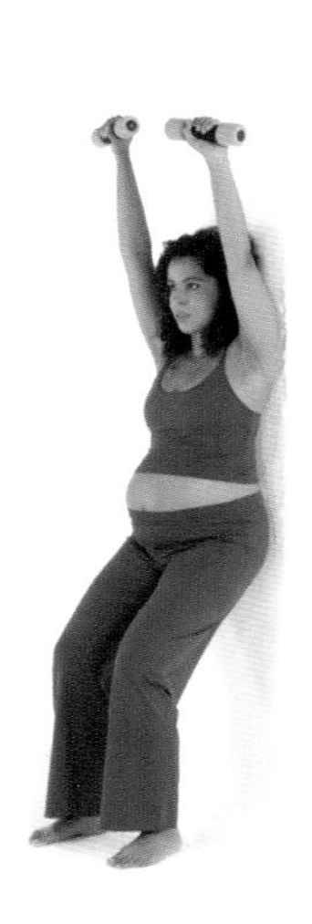
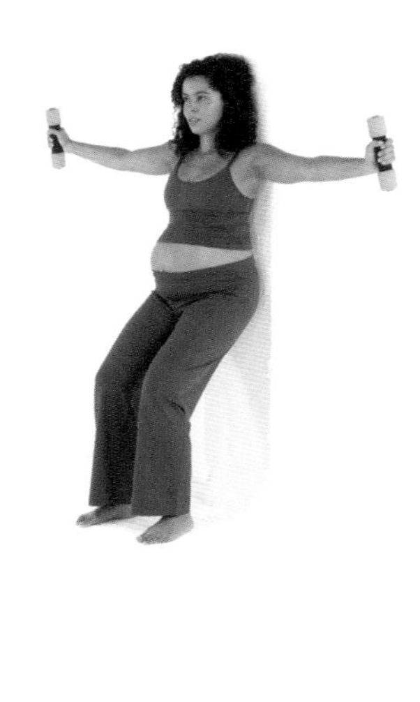
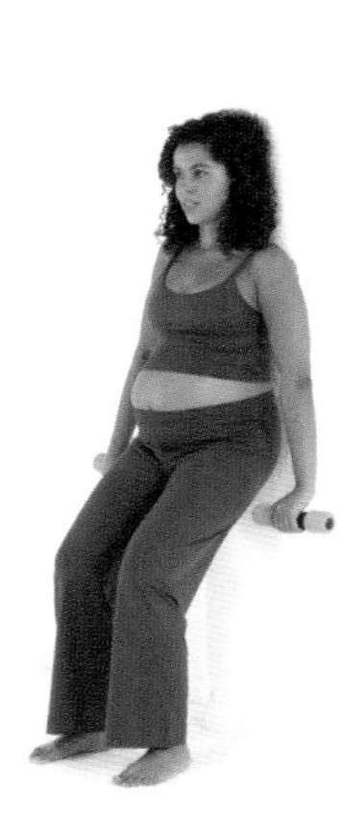

The Oyster

Probably not the most popular Body Control Pilates exercise, but it does hit the spot – deep in the buttocks!

Aim
To strengthen the gluteus medius muscle in the buttocks, which is a very important muscle for stabilizing the pelvis. This is also a very good exercise if you have knee problems.

Equipment
One or two cushions.

Starting Position
Lie on your side in a straight line. Have your underneath arm stretched out above your head in a line with your body, and place a flat cushion between your ear and your arm so your neck keeps in line with your spine. You can also put a cushion under your bump. Bend your knees, keeping your feet in a line with your bottom.

Action
1. Breathe in wide and full to prepare.
2. Breathe out, zip up and hollow and stay zipped and hollowed throughout. Slowly rotate your top leg, opening the knee. Make sure as you do so, that you do not lose your neutral pelvis or spine. Keep lengthening through the body. Your feet stay together on the floor. The action initiates in the buttock.
3. Breathe in and hold.
4. Breathe out and close.
5. Repeat 10 times on each side.

Watchpoints
- Do not allow the waist to sink into the floor; keep it long.
- Do not allow your upper body to fall forward.
- Maintain a neutral pelvis throughout.

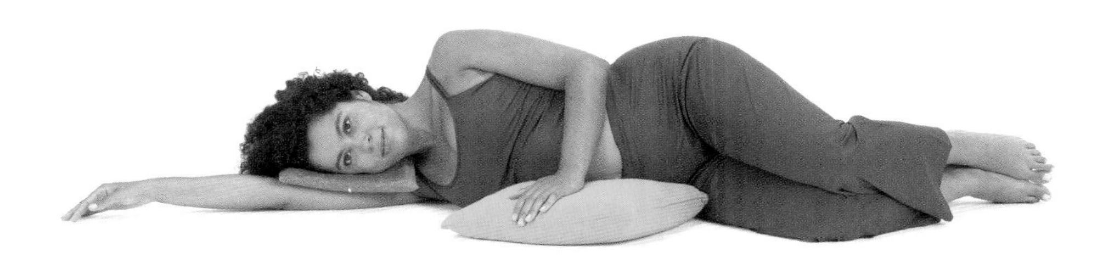

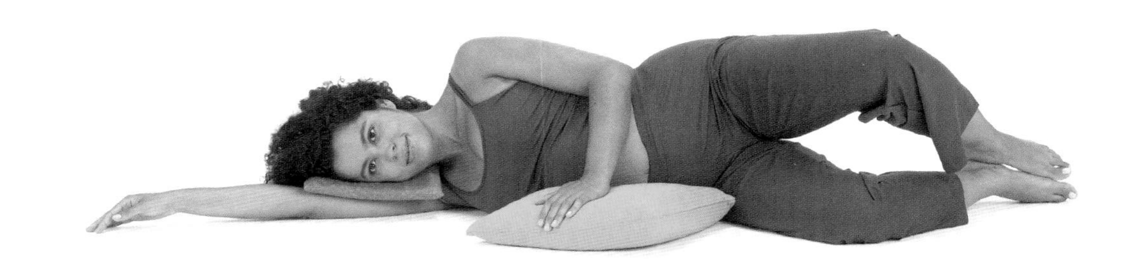

Pelvic Stability Check

It is a good idea to check your stability every now and then. This exercise does just that. Your pelvis should stay still.

Aim
To check the stability of your pelvis.

Starting Position
Lie in the Relaxation Position (page 26). Have your pelvis in neutral; it should remain in neutral throughout the exercise. Place your hands on your hip bones to check they stay still.

Action
1. Breathe in wide and full to prepare.
2. Breathe out, zip up and hollow, and fold one knee towards your chest, dropping the thigh bone down into the hip socket. Breathe in and check you are still in neutral.
3. Breathe out, still zipped, and extend the leg high into the air at an angle of about 45° to the floor. The pelvis stays still.
4. Breathe in as the leg bends in again, and out as you return the leg to the floor.
5. Repeat 3 times with each leg.

Watchpoints
- Keep both sides of your waist long.
- Don't forget that the upper body stays relaxed, breastbone soft, neck released.

IMPORTANT NOTE

You will need to change position regularly every 3 minutes if you are in your last two trimesters

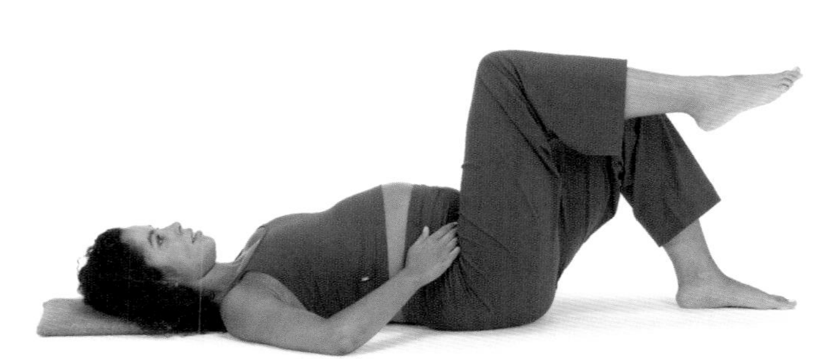

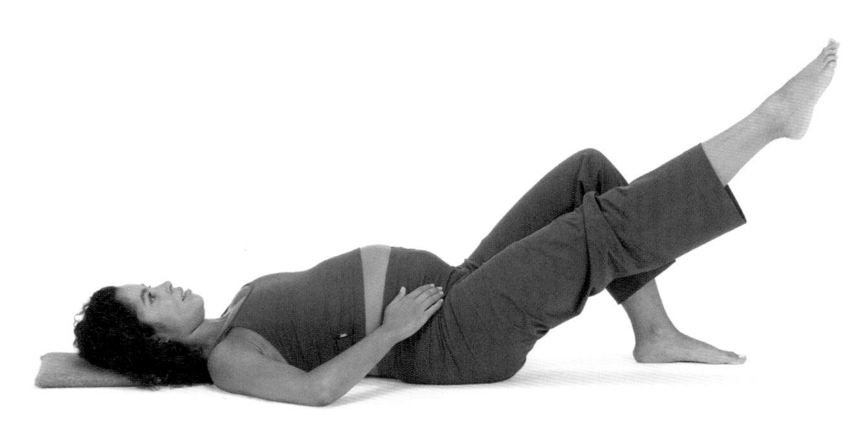

Chalk Circles

This exercise has the most wonderful feel-good factor. Perfect at the end of a bad day, or even a good day! You should be comfortable with Arm Openings (page 137) before you try it.

Equipment

3 pillows or large cushions.

Starting Position

Lie on your side, stacking your joints directly over each other. Place one pillow under your head – a bed pillow is perfect – another between your knees (keeping good alignment) and the third under your bump. Have your back in a straight line, but bend your knees up to hip level. Extend your arms in front of you, in line with your shoulders, palms together.

Action

1. Breathe in to prepare and lengthen through the spine.
2. Breathe out and zip up and hollow. Imagine you have a piece of chalk in your hand. Reach the top arm beyond the lower arm and move your hand up and round your head. Allow your head to move naturally, following the opening movement of the shoulders. The knees stay together and the centre strong. Do not over-reach.
3. Breathing normally, move your hand right around as if you are drawing a circle on the floor. It will pass behind you, down over your buttocks and back up to join the other hand.
4. Repeat 5 times on each side. The aim is to keep the hand in contact with the floor but, if that's difficult, please work within your comfort range.

Watchpoints

- As you allow your head to follow the movement, take care that you do not shorten the back of the neck – it should stay released.
- Keep the waist long but do not allow the back to arch.
- Keep the knees on the ground, even if it means that your hand does not touch the floor.
- Do not force the arm at all.

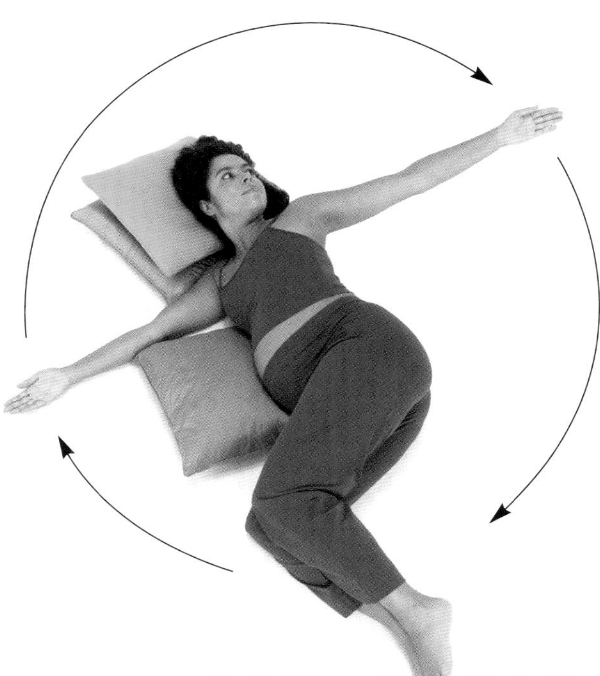

Pole Raises

Add this exercise to your workout when you are feeling as though you need more space inside. This exercise is often done using a pole (hence the name) but can also be done with a scarf or stretchband.

Aim
To learn correct upper body use. To open the upper body.

Equipment
A long scarf or a pole.

Starting Position
Stand tall. Focus on your three body weights balancing and floating over each other. Lengthen up through the spine. Hold the scarf or pole lightly, with both hands about one metre (3 feet) apart.

Action

1. Breathe in wide and full to prepare.
2. Breathe out and zip up and hollow as you raise the scarf, allowing the movement of the hands and the scarf to lead the arms and shoulders. Try to keep the upper shoulders relaxed – don't let them hike up around your ears. Think of the shoulder blades dropping down as the arms rise. Make the movement initiate from your shoulder blades.
3. Breathe in.
4. Breathe out as you bring the scarf or pole on to your forehead, bringing the shoulder blades down into your back as you do so.
5. Breathe in and raise the scarf or pole.
6. Breathe out and slowly lower the scarf or pole using those muscles below the shoulder blades.
7. Repeat 3 times.

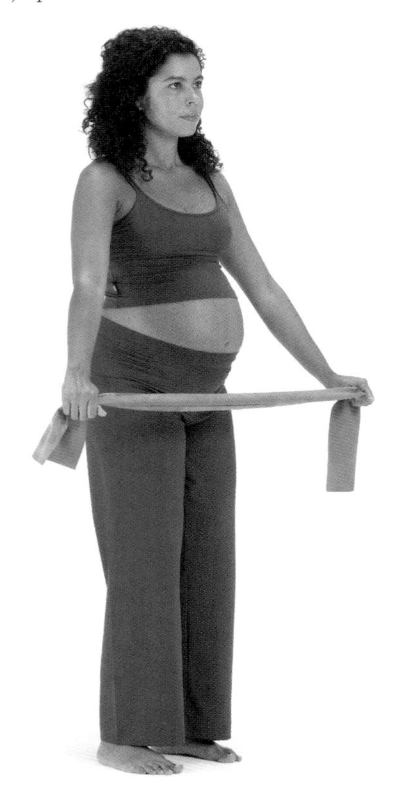

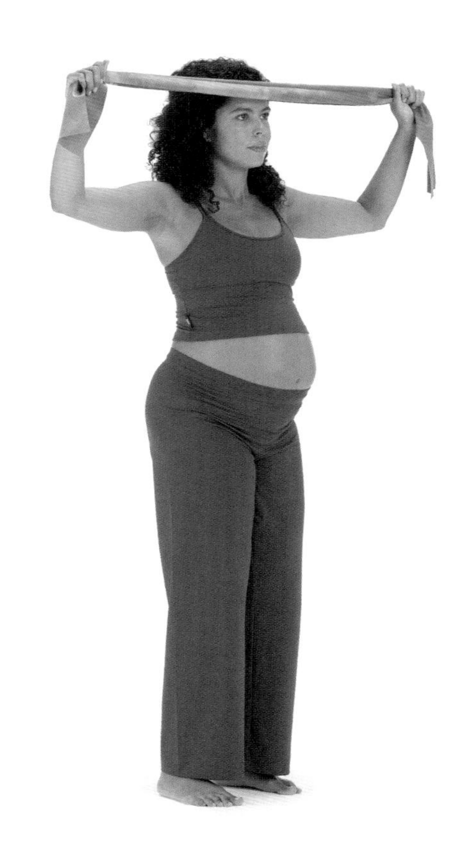

Moving on . . . when you are comfortable with this movement, follow directions 1–3 then:

1. Breathe out and bring the scarf or pole directly down behind you, keeping it close to your body and bending the elbows, so that you have a chicken-wing shape. Think of the shoulder blades drawing down and together.
2. Breathe in as you slowly raise the scarf or pole from behind. Breathe out, as you bring it back down in front slowly.
3. Repeat up to 3 times.

Watchpoints

- As the arms rise, try to keep the ribcage calm.
- Do not allow the back to arch – keep the neutral spine alignment; keep your head, ribcage and pelvis balanced over each other.
- Try not to duck your head as the scarf or pole comes over. Try to keep both the shoulders and the arms moving together – don't allow one shoulder to dominate.
- Keep reminding yourself of the instructions for Standing Well (page 16), and lengthen the spine upwards.

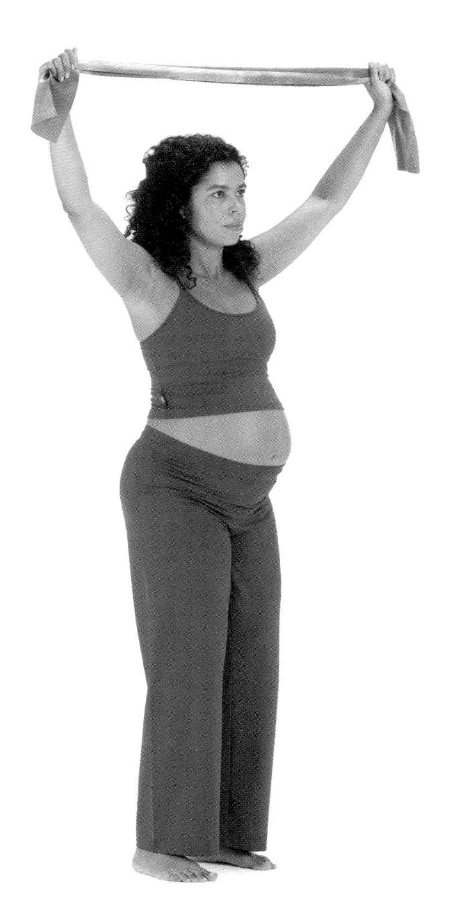

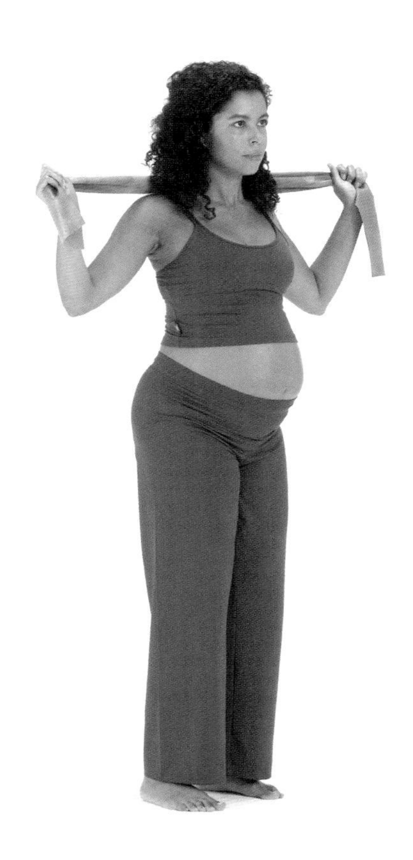

Tennis Ball Rises

This is another way to include squatting in your workout. Even this small movement opens the pelvic outlet. This exercise is great for learning good body alignment. Once again, those three body weights – head, ribcage and pelvis – need to be properly balanced over each other. It's also a calf stretch so it works the calf pump and helps circulation in the legs. A good all rounder!

Aim
To learn good alignment of the body, feet, ankles, knees and hips. To strengthen the quadriceps, to stretch the Achilles tendon and calves. To work the stabilizing muscles of the knee, especially vastus medialis.

Equipment
Two tennis balls, or one tennis ball and a small cushion.

Starting Position
Stand sideways on to a wall or by a sturdy chair, and place the tennis ball between your ankles, just below your inside ankle bone. Place another tennis ball or a small cushion between the thighs just above the knees. Remind yourself of all the directions for Standing Well (page 16). Hold on to the wall or the chair.

Action

1. Breathe in and lengthen up through the spine – imagine someone is pulling you up from the top of your head, but that there is also a weight on your tailbone, anchoring your spine. Breathe out, zip up and hollow, and rise up on to your toes.
2. Breathe in.
3. Breathe out, and slowly lengthen your heels back down to the floor. Imagine that your head stays up.
4. When your heels are on the floor, slightly bend your knees directly over your feet on the out breath, keeping the heels down. Do not allow your bottom to stick out.
5. Breathe in and return.
6. Repeat 6 times.

Watchpoints

- Keep the heels on the ground as you bend the knees.
- Keep the weight evenly balanced on the feet.
- Keep lengthening upwards throughout.

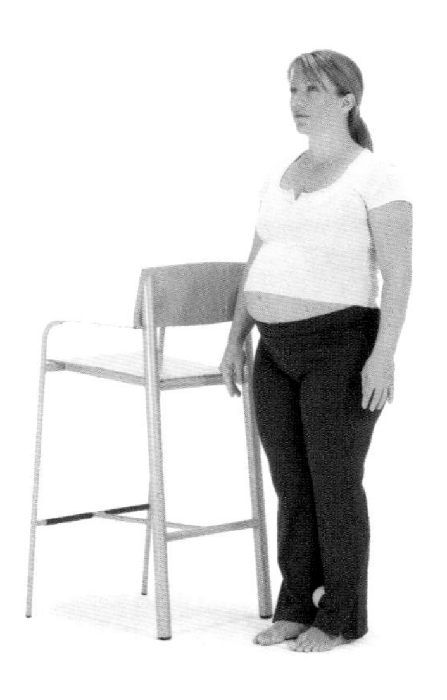

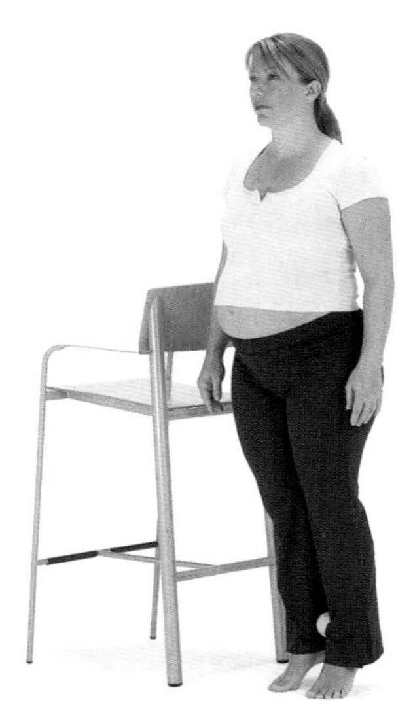

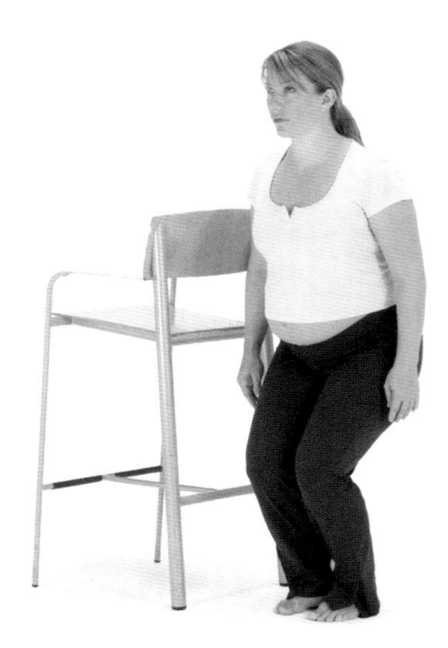

The Cat

A wonderful exercise to help you feel how to move the spine bone by bone. Four-point kneeling should feel great, as it takes the weight of the baby off the spine. As you zip up and hollow in this position you have to lift your bump against gravity – your own built-in training weight!

If you suffer from carpal tunnel syndrome, or even if you just find this position hard on your wrists, rest the heels of your hands on a rolled-up towel; it will lessen the angle at the wrist.

Aim
To mobilize the spine and learn correct alignment.

Equipment
A towel (optional).

Starting Position
Kneel on all fours. Place your hands directly beneath your shoulders, with the fingers facing forwards. You may like to rest the heels of your hands on a towel. Your knees should be in line with your hips, the lower legs straight. Look straight down at the floor so that the back of your neck is long. Find the natural, neutral curve in your spine. Think of a small pool of water in the small of your back. Keep lengthening the top of your head away from your tailbone. Your shoulder blades should be down into your back. Do not be tempted to lock your elbows. Keep your weight on the whole of the hand, not just the heels.

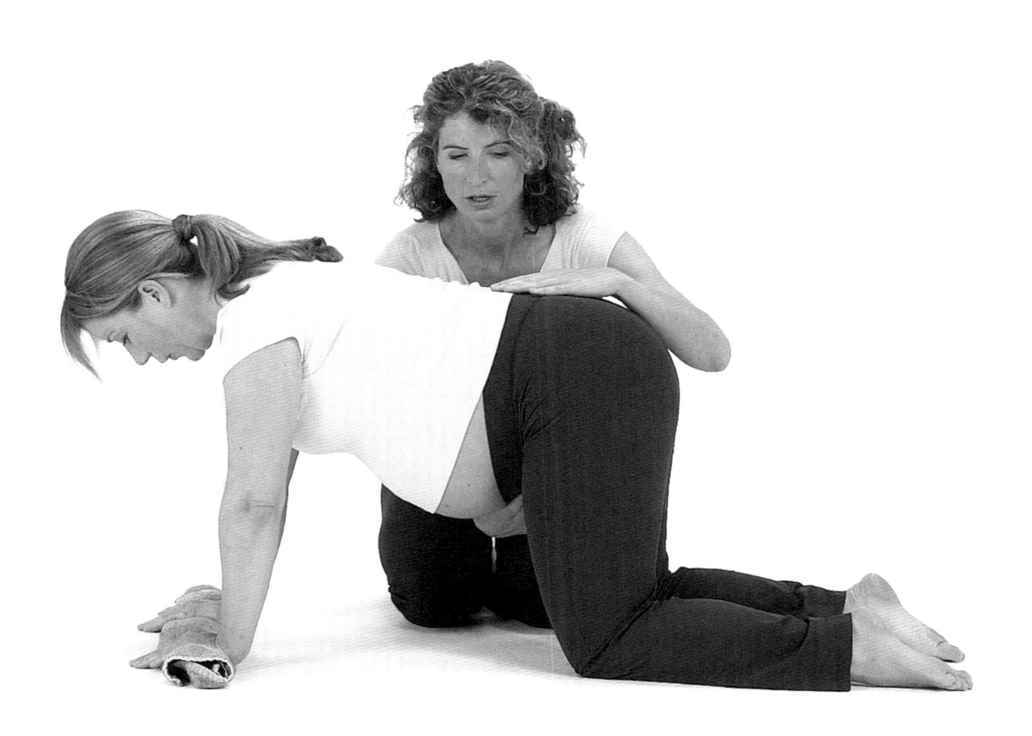

Action

1. Breathe in wide and full to prepare and lengthen through the spine.
2. Breathe out, zip up and hollow and stay zipped and hollowed throughout. Starting with the base of the spine, start to curl your tailbone under – a bit like you did for Spine Curls (page 67). Work your way up your back, rounding it, but keeping it open and wide. Your chin will end up on your chest; neck and head released.
3. Breathe in wide, checking that your elbows haven't locked.
4. Breathe out, and slowly uncurl the spine starting again from the base, sticking your tailbone out, mobilizing vertebra by vertebra, sliding the shoulder blades down into your back, until you have returned to the Starting Position, i.e. neutral. Please do not over-dip the low back or lift the head back. Feel the length of the spine.
5. Repeat 5 times.

Watchpoints

- Keep the weight even on both hands.
- If your wrists tire, stop for a short break, then start again. Eventually they will strengthen.
- Focus on moving the spine bone by bone.
- Do not lock your elbows!
- Stop at neutral when you return to the Starting Position – do not overarch the low back.
- Do not hunch your shoulders up around your ears.

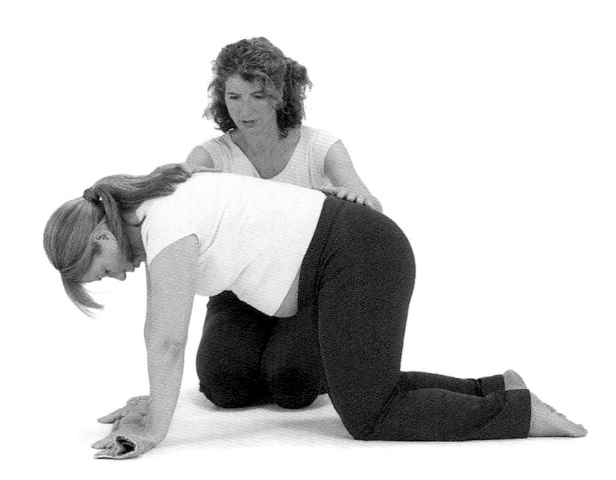

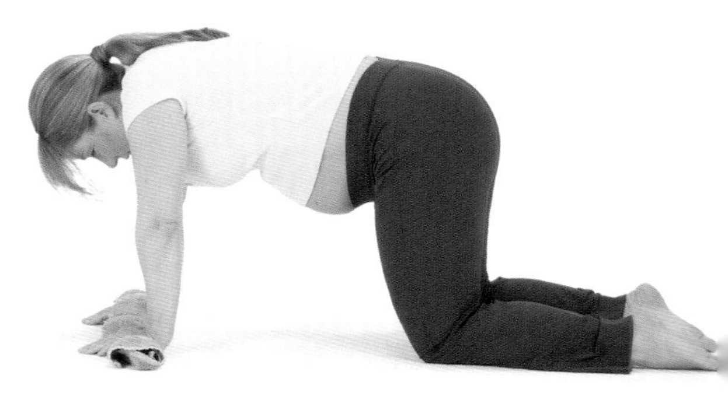

✕ **Do not hunch your shoulders**

Standing or Sitting Tarzan

A fun exercise which targets the biceps.
All the better for carrying baby with!

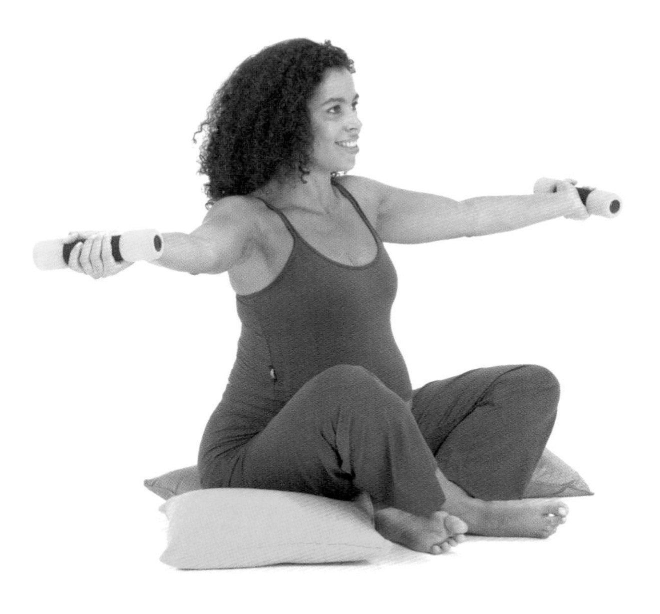

Equipment
Light hand-held weights of up to 1 kilo (2 pounds) each weight.

Starting Position
Stand or sit correctly. Hold your arms out to the sides, palms up, shoulder blades down into your back, neck released. Have the arms straight but not locked.

Action
1. Breathe in wide and full and lengthen up through the spine.
2. Breathe out, zip up and hollow and stay gently zipped and hollowed throughout. Slowly curl your arms in, hingeing from the elbows.
3. Breathe in and slowly straighten the arm again.
4. Repeat 6 times.

Watchpoints
- Keep the upper arm quite still.
- As you straighten the arms think of lengthening away.
- Lower your arms if they feel tired.

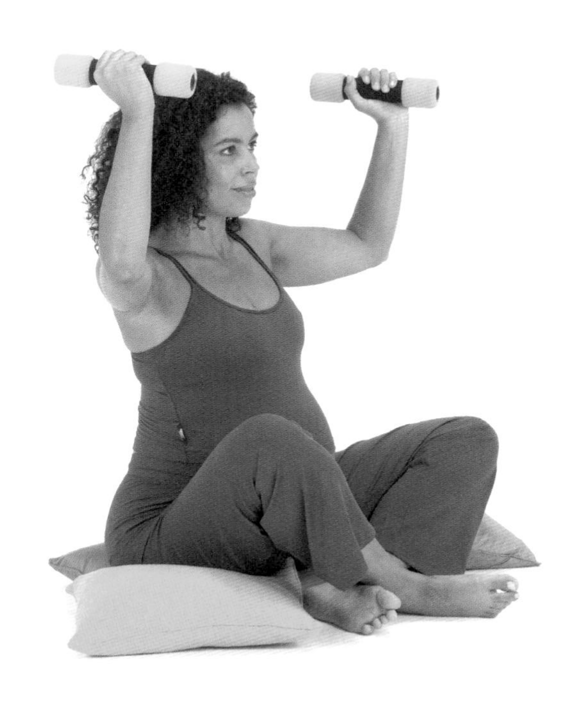

Back Press

Another good arm and upper-back strengthener. This exercise can also be done without weights.

Equipment
Hand-held weights of 0.5 kilo (1 pound) each weight.

Starting Position
Stand correctly, with your arms relaxed and down by your sides, palms facing backwards. Hold the weights in each hand.

Action
1. Breathe in wide and lengthen through the spine.
2. Breathe out and zip up and hollow.
3. Breathe in and press your arms back, opening the chest but not allowing the upper back to arch or the ribcage to flare.
4. Breathe out and release.
5. Repeat 6 times.

Watchpoints
- Keeping good alignment through the body is essential in this exercise. It is very easy to tip the upper body forward. Use your core muscles to keep you upright, head balanced over ribcage, ribcage over pelvis.
- Keep your neck released.
- Try not to squeeze between the shoulder blades.
- Keep the distance between your ears and your shoulders.

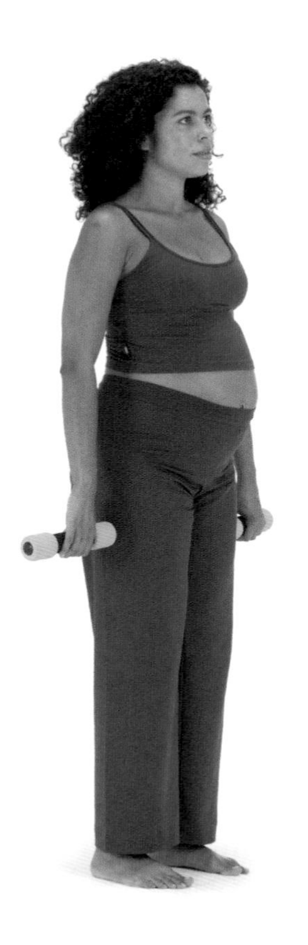

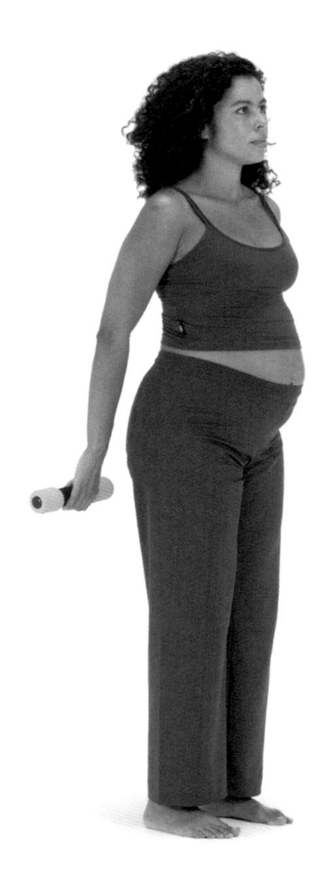

Pelvic Floor Release

Essential preparation for the birth itself. Make sure that your bladder is empty before practising release work . . . just in case!

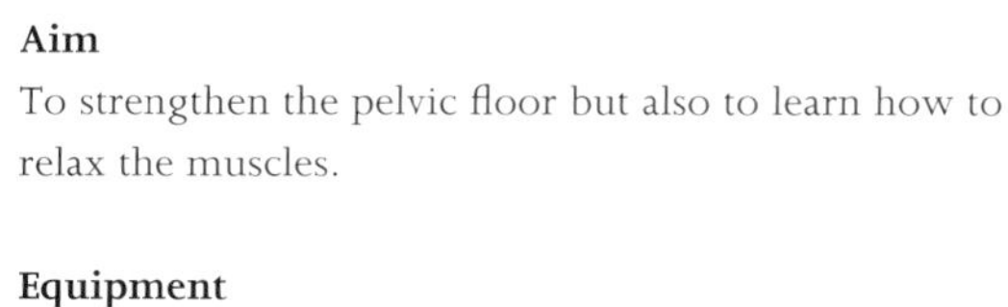

Aim
To strengthen the pelvic floor but also to learn how to relax the muscles.

Equipment
A sturdy chair or a physio ball.

Action
1. Sit up tall on a chair or physio ball.
2. Start practising the Pelvic Elevator (page 70), but when you take the lift back down to the ground floor, don't stop there. Let it go completely down to the basement!
3. Return to the ground floor and start again.
4. Repeat 6 times.

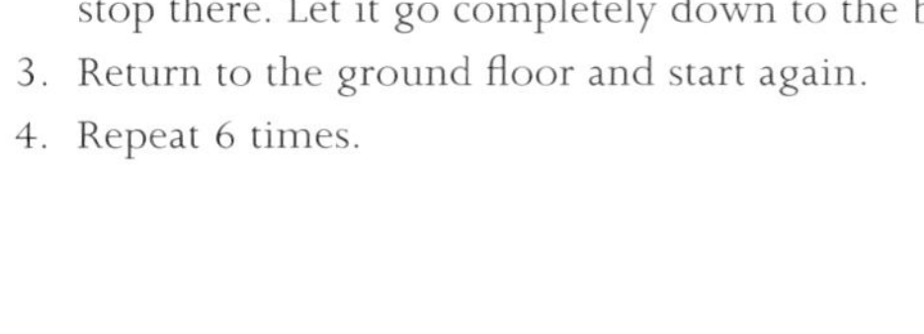

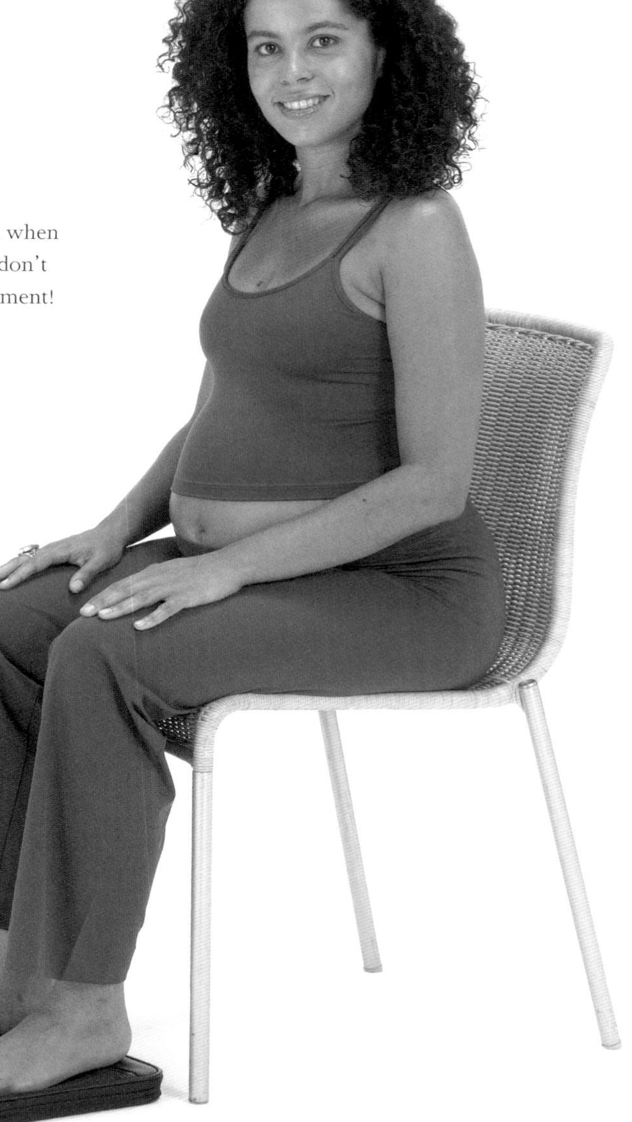

The Flower

Aim
To strengthen the pelvic floor but also to learn how to relax and release the muscles.

Equipment
A sturdy chair or a physio ball.

Action
Sit on the chair or physio ball. Gradually draw the pelvic floor up and in, just like a flower closing at the end of the day. Now, gradually release the muscles, letting them open like a flower opening in the morning sun. Then gently close the flower again.

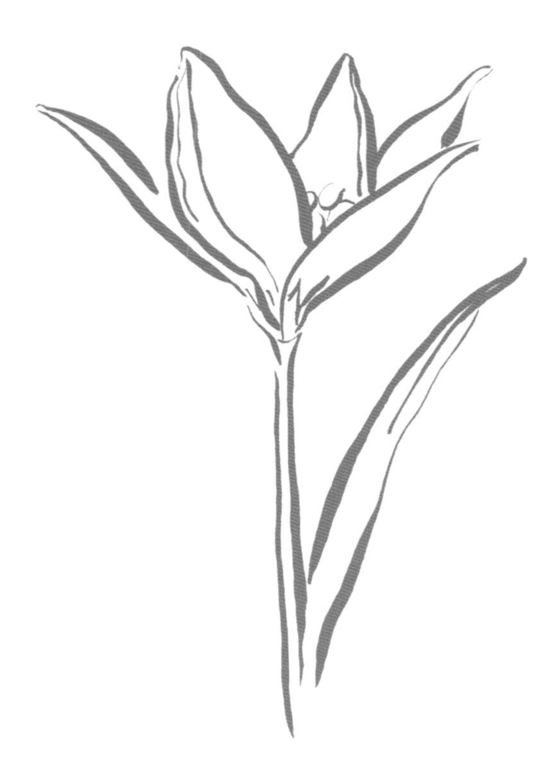

The Scapular Squeeze

A wonderful exercise for the upper back and the upper arms where, unfortunately, we all tend to get a bit flabby! Not any more, if you do this exercise and all the exercises using arm weights!

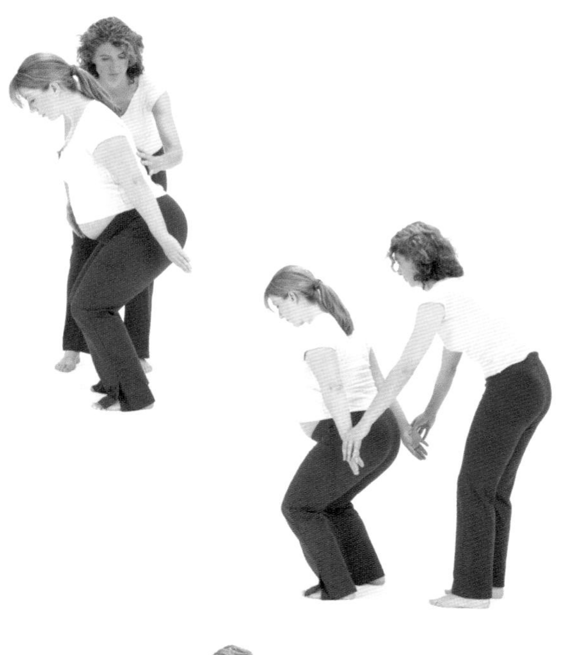

Aim

To strengthen the stabilizing muscles between and underneath the shoulder blades, opening the chest. To strengthen the back of the upper arms. To lengthen the spine.

Starting Position

Stand, feet in parallel, hip-width apart. Your knees are bent directly over your feet. Now pivot forward on your hips as if you are skiing downhill, your head, neck and back remain in one piece. Look at a spot on the floor in front of you at a distance that keeps the back of your neck free from tension and the top of your head lengthening away (see photo). If you look too closely, your head will drop; too far away and you shorten the back of the neck. Take your arms behind you and to the sides. The palms face upwards.

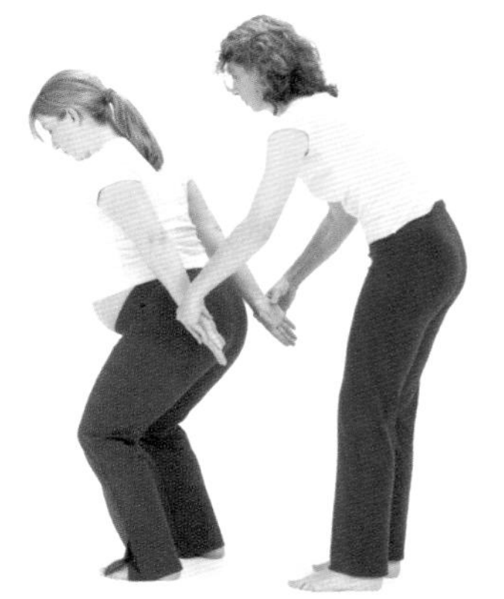

Action

1. Breathe in to prepare and lengthen up through the spine.
2. Breathe out, zip up and hollow, and slide the shoulder blades down before you squeeze them together. Your arms are also squeezing towards each other as if the thumbs want to meet.
3. Breathe in and hold.
4. Breathe out, and release the arms.
5. Repeat 5 times before returning to upright.
6. When coming back to upright, keep lengthening your back and head away and return to a balanced way of standing without locking your knees.

Watchpoints

- Keep your gaze on your spot on the floor.
- Check your neck – keep it released and long.
- Think of the tailbone lengthening downwards and away from the top of your head.
- Keep the knees softly bent and over your feet.
- Make sure you feel this exercise between the shoulder blades and also at the back of your upper arms. Do not lock the arms – they are straight but not locked.

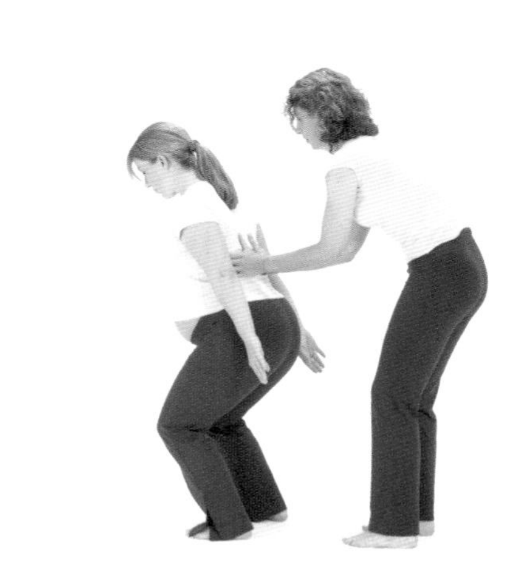

Adductor Openings

It does not need a great deal of imagination to appreciate why this exercise is a useful preparation for delivery!

Empty your bladder before doing a pelvic release.

IMPORTANT NOTE

You will need to change position regularly every 3 minutes if you are in your last two trimesters

Aim

To gently stretch the inner thighs – the adductors.
To practise pelvic floor release.

Starting Position

Lie in the Relaxation Position (page 26).

Action

1. Breathe in wide and full to prepare.
2. Breathe out, zip up and hollow, and bring one knee at a time on to your chest in a Double Knee Fold (page 74).
3. Breathing normally, place one hand under each knee and allow the legs to open slowly. This will stretch your inner thighs. Hold this position for 2 minutes only – watch the clock. Do not allow your back to arch. If you like, you can practise a pelvic floor release by doing the Flower (page 160) at the same time.
4. After 2 minutes, slowly close the legs and return your feet one by one to the floor, while zipping up and hollowing.

Watchpoint

- Stay in neutral.

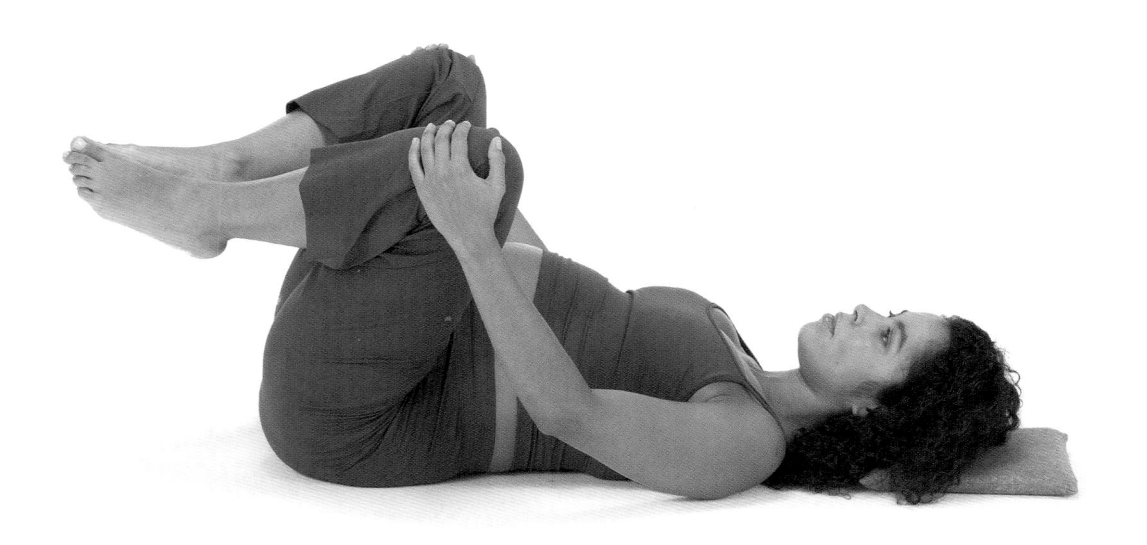

Squatting

Squatting is a popular birth position. When you squat, the pelvis is wide open and the baby's head is pressing down. If you can practise in the last few weeks it will feel more natural and comfortable during the birth itself. Have your partner help you. You may not be able to get back up again otherwise!

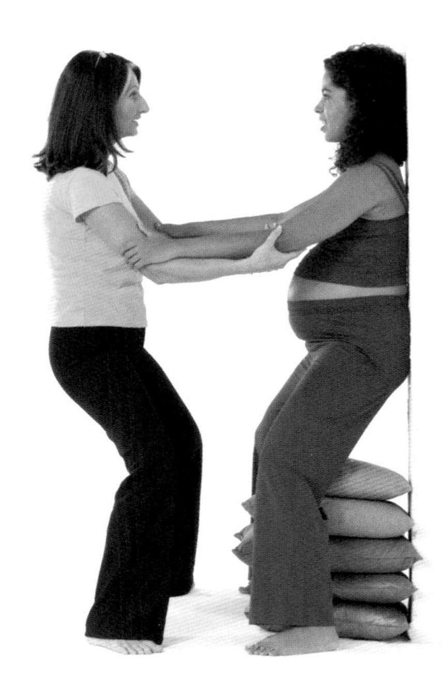

Equipment
Several large, soft pillows and a towel.

Action with a Partner

1. With your back to a wall, place a pile of pillows underneath you.
2. Face each other with your feet naturally turned out just a little. Hold each other's forearms firmly.
3. Breathe in wide and, as you breathe out, zip up and stay zipped and slowly lower down into a squat. Breathe normally. Your heels may come off the floor. If they do, you can place a rolled-up towel under them.
4. Try to direct your knees over the centre of your feet. Think of lengthening from your tailbone to the top of your head. Don't stay too long in this position.
5. You will need strong thighs to come up from a squat. Come up slowly, still zipping. Keep thinking of length through the spine.

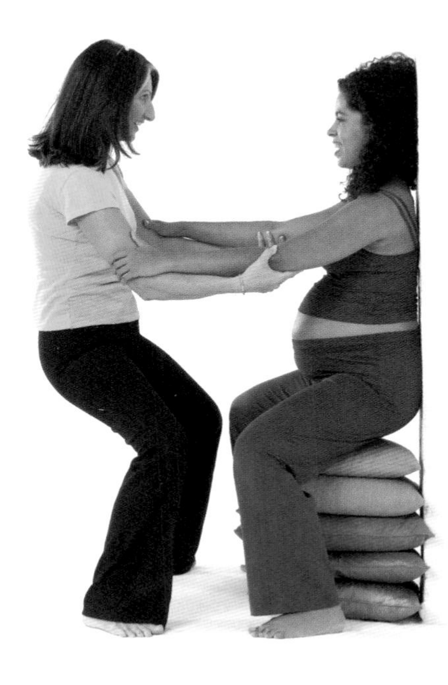

NOTE

Squatting may place a lot of strain on the knees so avoid this if you have knee problems. Stop if you feel any knee discomfort.

Squatting with a Partner

You can also try squatting away from a wall, but you will need a partner. If a full squat is uncomfortable, you could try a sitting squat. Place a folded towel on a low stool and sit with the legs wide in a half squatting position. This is a very good position to practise your pelvic floor releases.

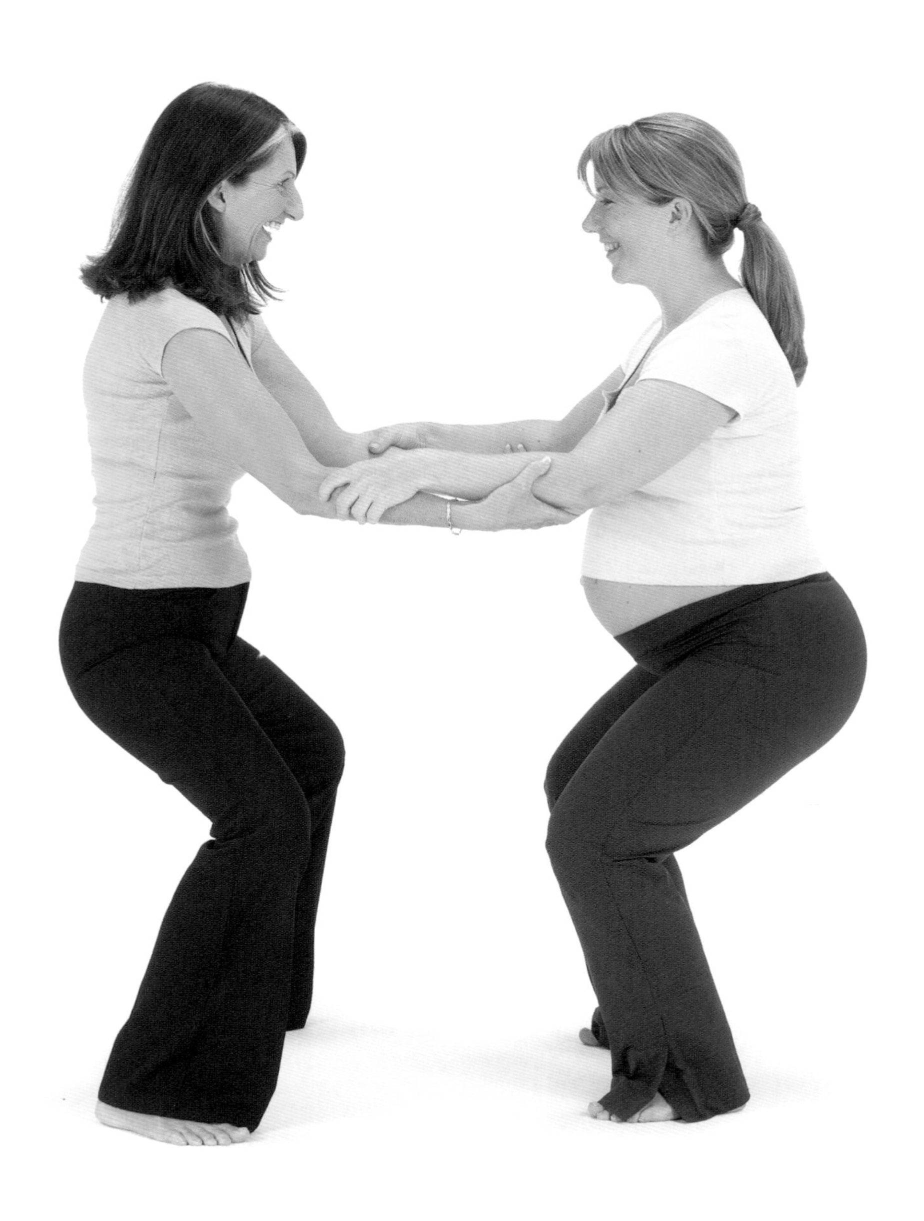

Relaxation

Learning to relax will not only help you through your pregnancy, but will also help during the birth process. Babies, before they are born as well as after, thrive in a calm, relaxed environment. The body needs time to unwind and slow down after working, exercising and socializing. Sometimes it takes more than a hot drink and 5 minutes with your feet up to feel completely relaxed.

For the following relaxation, see if you can get a friend (preferably one with a lovely, deep, sexy voice) to record the directions on to tape. Eliminate distractions and interruptions such as the phone, radio, television and other people. Make sure the room is warm, softly lit (candles are ideal) and cosy.

Normally, we would recommend that you do this in the Relaxation Position (page 26), but as you will be in the same position for some time, you will need to adapt the position so you are not lying flat on your back. Pile up as many cushions and pillows as you can against a wall. A sloping piece of foam would be ideal. You should try to keep your body symmetrical and your back supported. Put some more pillows under your knees. You might like to on your left side or try using the belly bag, or perhaps get into the Rest Position (page 93) (using lots of cushions). For all these positions you will have to adapt the direction accordingly.

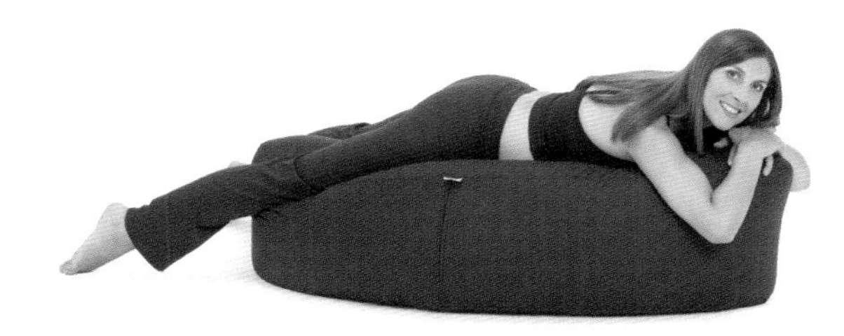

Directions

1. Take your awareness down to your feet and soften the soles, uncurling the toes.
2. Soften your ankles.
3. Soften your calves.
4. Release your knees.
5. Release your thighs.
6. Allow your hips to open.
7. Allow the small of your back to sink into the floor as though you are sinking down into the folds of a hammock.
8. Feel the length of your spine.
9. Take your awareness down to your hands, stretch your fingers away from your palms, feel the centre of your palms opening.
10. Allow the fingers to curl, the palms to soften.
11. Allow your elbows to open and the front of your shoulders to soften.
12. With each out-breath allow your shoulder blades to widen.
13. Allow your breastbone to soften.
14. Allow your neck to release.
15. Check your jaw; it should be loose and free.
16. Allow your tongue to widen at its base and rest comfortably at the bottom of your mouth.
17. Your lips are softly closed.
18. Your eyes are softly closed.
19. Your forehead is wide and smooth and completely free of lines.
20. Your face feels soft.
21. Your body feels soft and warm.
22. Your spine is gently released down into the floor.
23. Observe your breathing, but do not interrupt it, simply enjoy its natural rhythm.

To Come Out of the Relaxation

1. Very gently allow your head to roll to one side, allowing its own weight to move it. Slowly come back to the centre and allow it to roll to the other side, then bring it back to the centre.
2. Wriggle your fingers . . . and then your toes.
3. When you are ready, move out of your chosen relaxation position slowly and thoughtfully.

Third Trimester Workouts

There are 5 balanced workouts set out below. Each lasts approximately 20–30 minutes, and you should try to do all 5 workouts once each week.

The exercises are mainly drawn from this chapter but we have also added a few from earlier chapters which will make the workouts more varied.

The workouts are designed so that you change position frequently. You may need to cut the number of repetitions that you do if you have spent more than 3 minutes lying on your back.

Workout One

The Full Starfish 65
The Oyster 149
Baby Spine Curls with Pillow Squeeze 123
Chalk Circles 151
Pelvic Stability Check 150
Chest Expansion 131
Adductor Openings 162
The Pelvic Elevator, Pelvic Floor Release, the Flower 70, 159, 160
Tennis Ball Rises 154
Pole Raises 152
Bow and Arrow 126
Ankle Circles 112
The Cat 155
The Pillow Squeeze 127
Squatting 163
Walking on the Spot 124

Workout Two

Sliding Down the Wall 135
The Corkscrew 125
Baby Spine Curls with Pillow Squeeze 123
Side-lying Circles 134
Windows 132
The Cat 155
Shoulder Drops 66
Sitting Side Reach 86
Pelvic Floor Release and Emergency Stop 159 and 71
The Dumb Waiter 101
Standing or Sitting Tarzan 157
The Scapular Squeeze 160
Bow and Arrow 126
The Full Starfish 65

Workout Three

Monkey Bends with Arms 129
Arm Circles Against the Wall 148
Walking on the Spot 124
Pelvic Stability Check 150
The Oyster 149
Hip Rolls (Level One only) 81
Sliding Down the Wall 135
Sitting Side Reach 86
Ankle Circles 112
Bow and Arrow 126
Pelvic Floor Release 159
Calf Stretch 130
Squatting 163
Back Press 158
Chest Expansion 131
Pillow Squeeze 127

Workout Four

Monkey Bends with Arms 129
The Cat 155
Baby Spine Curls with Pillow Squeeze 123
Chalk Circles 157
Shoulder Drops 66
Abductor and Adductor Lifts (no weights) 87 and 89
Adductor Openings 162
Chest Expansion 131
Scapular Squeeze 160
Pole Raises 152
Pelvic Floor Release 159
Sitting Side Reach 86
Ankle Circles 112
Bow and Arrow 126
Squatting 163

Workout Five

Tennis Ball Rises 154
The Dumb Waiter 101
The Corkscrew 125
Sitting Side Reach 86
Pillow Squeeze 127
Side-lying Circles 134
Windows 132
Bow and Arrow 126
Pelvic Floor Release 159
The Cat 155
Pelvic Stability Check 150
Arm Openings 137
Back Press 158
Arm Circles Against the Wall 148
Monkey Bends with Arms 129

Pilates was tremendous for my posture, strength and keeping me toned during my pregnancy. I would highly recommend it!

– Kate Mills

10 The First Six Weeks After the Birth

Congratulations! You are a mum!

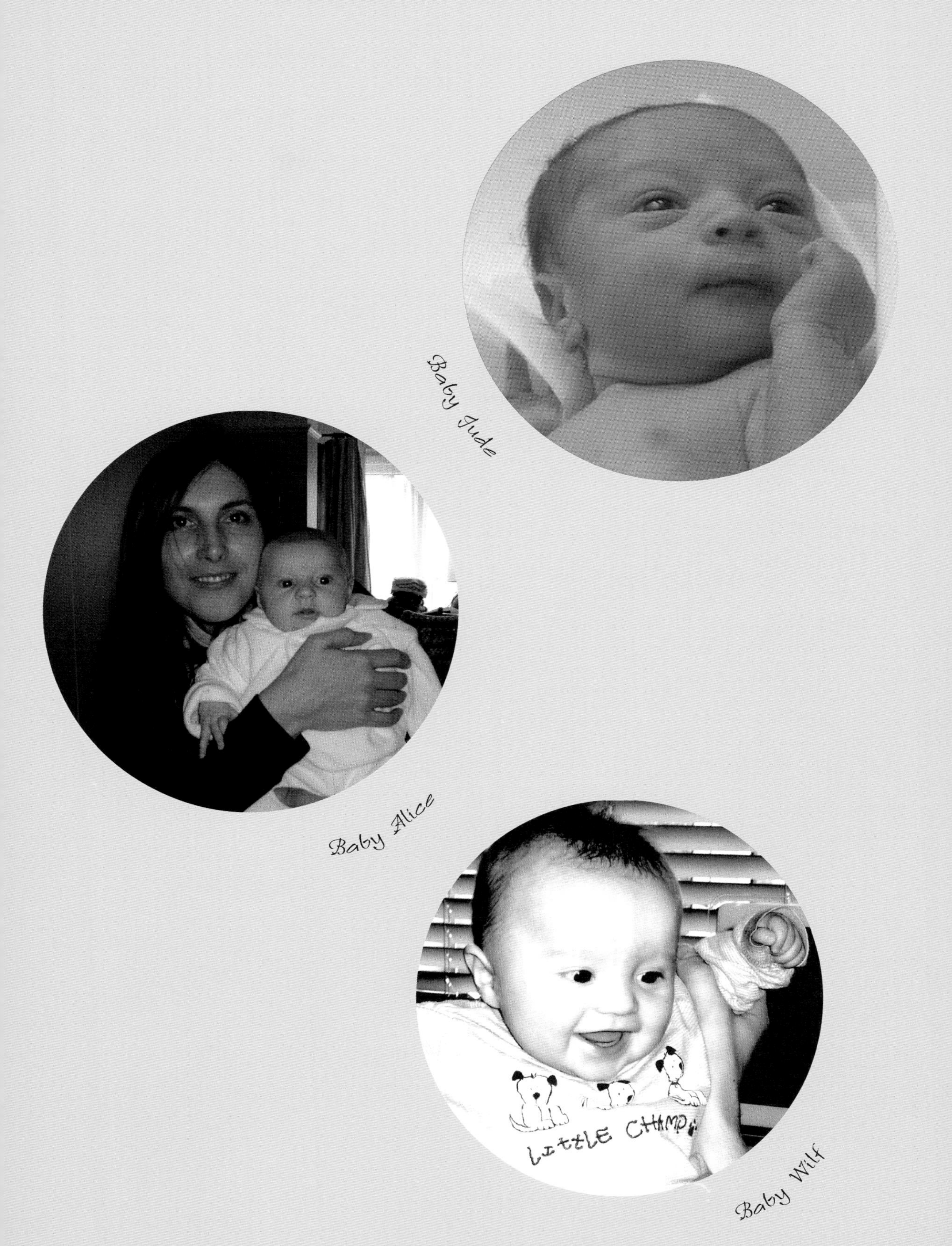

Baby Jude

Baby Alice

Baby Wilf

Normal Deliveries

The advice we are going to give over the next few pages relates to a mother who has had a normal delivery. If you had a caesarean section, please turn to page 174.

Naturally your main focus is now going to be on your baby and rightly so . . . but it is essential you put time aside to look after yourself. The fitter, healthier and more relaxed you are, the better mum you will be. Looking back over the previous chapters you can see the multitude of ways in which your body changed as your pregnancy progressed. You had time to adjust to these changes. Now, however, after the birth, your body is changing again, but rapidly; you will start to produce breast milk, for example. You may also experience a roller coaster of emotions from high to low. It will take a lot of discipline to do your exercises, but if you can, you will be taking important steps towards recovery from the delivery and regaining your former pre-pregnancy shape.

Obviously, you are going to feel tired and sore for the first few days after the birth. Your uterus usually takes about 6 weeks to return to its normal size, this is called involution. And to begin with you will feel after-pains as a result of the uterus contracting and from the hormone oxytoxin, which is produced when you put the baby to your breast. The pains are strongest while you are breast feeding. They usually last just a few days and are accompanied by a discharge known as lochia, which is the shedding of the lining of the uterus. To help, as soon as you can, you should try some very small Baby Spine Curls (page 123).

Your pelvic floor is going to feel sore after the delivery. The pressure of the baby's head passing through the vagina will probably have bruised the area and you may have stitches from a tear or an episiotomy (a cut sometimes made to enlarge the vagina opening during delivery). You will probably feel the need to empty your bladder frequently while your body rids itself of the extra fluid you carried during pregnancy. If you had an epidural during labour then you may have had a catheter fitted to help, because you may not yet have normal sensation in that region. It is possible that you will find passing urine difficult and you may also suffer from stress incontinence – where you will pass urine involuntarily whenever extra pressure is created inside the abdomen, for example when you cough or sneeze. If you did your pelvic floor exercises regularly throughout your pregnancy you will be less likely to suffer from this.

The last thing you probably feel like doing at this stage is pelvic floor exercises – you may think that they will aggravate the stitches, but in fact the opposite is true. These exercises tighten and relax the muscles and thus encourage the flow of blood to the area, which helps the healing process. You should start your pelvic floor exercises 24 hours after the birth.

IMPORTANT NOTE

You must get your midwife to give you the go-ahead to start exercising again.

Pelvic Floor Exercises

A reminder:

- Pelvic floor exercises are best done in frequent batches of about 6 contractions at a time.
- Try to focus on drawing up every muscle fibre – it is the quality of the contraction that counts.
- Never hold your breath while contracting the pelvic floor.
- Try to do your pelvic floor exercises regularly throughout the day – while waiting at traffic lights, while queuing, etc. You can do these exercises in any position which is comfortable.

The Pelvic Elevator

Repeat the directions on page 70, but do not take the lift to the basement.

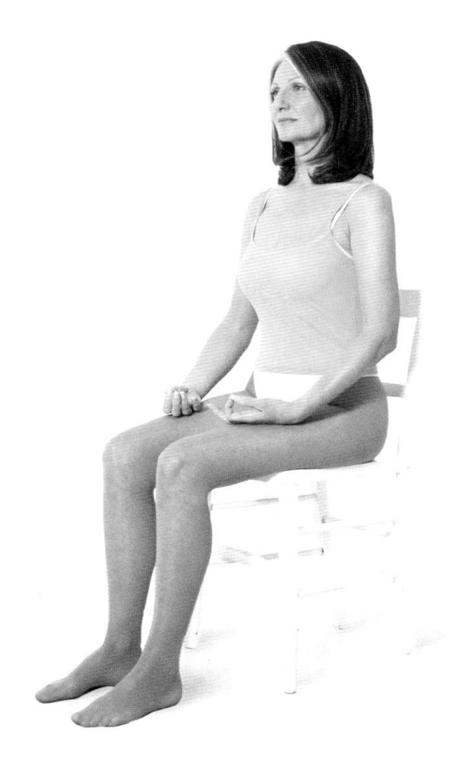

Figure of Eight

Equipment
A sturdy, hard-backed chair. A cushion (optional).

Starting Position
Sit squarely on a chair with your feet hip-width apart and flat on the floor (use a cushion under them if necessary). Check that your pelvis is in neutral, your spine long and your shoulders relaxed.

Action
1. Take your awareness down to your pelvic floor.
2. Breathe out and try to close the urethra (the front passage from which you pass urine).
3. Breathe in and check that your shoulders are still relaxed.
4. Breathe out and, still lifting from the front, try to close the muscles around the anus (back passage) keeping your buttocks relaxed!
5. Breathe in, and double check that your shoulders and jaw are soft.
6. Breathe out, and add lifting from the vagina, holding all three openings.
7. Then slowly release.

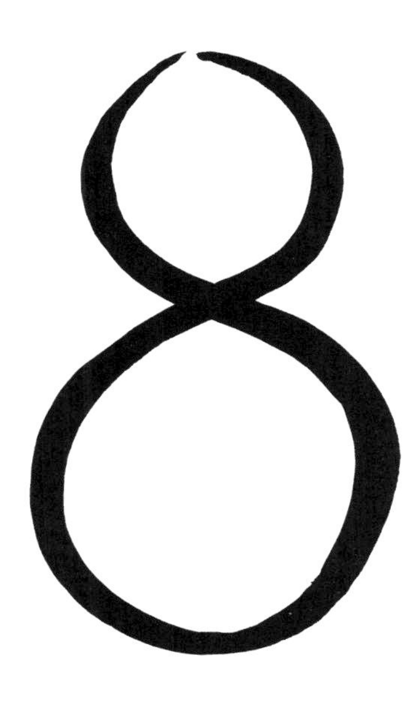

The Emergency Stop

Stress incontinence is very common after the delivery. The following exercises will help you to cope with emergencies such as coughing or sneezing.

Equipment
A sturdy, hard-backed chair. A cushion (optional).

Starting Position
Sit squarely on a chair with your feet hip-width apart and flat on the floor (use a cushion under them if necessary). Check that your pelvis is in neutral, your spine long and your shoulders relaxed.

Action
1. Simply lift the whole of the pelvic floor, tightening it all quickly as if in an emergency. Hold for about 5 seconds, then release. Keep breathing.
2. Repeat 5 times.

Sometimes with a difficult delivery, for example a forceps delivery, there may be some nerve damage which will make engaging these muscles difficult. If, after several weeks you are still experiencing stress incontinence or if you simply cannot make that connection with the pelvic floor muscle, do ask your GP for help. Do not suffer in silence. Occasionally an operation is needed to repair the vaginal wall, or electrical stimulation can help reactivate the muscles. Far better to get this sorted out now, than suffer long term. A stitch in time!!

If you felt that passing urine was difficult, this is nothing compared to passing your first bowel movement! It is really important that you avoid constipation and straining as this puts pressure on the pelvic floor. Drinking plenty of water, moving around, eating fibre-rich foods and doing your pelvic floor exercises will help because they improve circulation in the area.

The exercises listed below are perfectly safe for you to try when you feel able to do them so long as you have had a normal delivery with no complications. You will need to check with your doctor or midwife who can advise you. Don't feel that you need to do the whole workout at one time – far better to do a few exercises precisely and with control. Even 10 minutes will give you some benefits. If any exercise causes you discomfort, stop immediately.

It's very important that you get on to and up from the mat correctly in these early weeks. Follow the directions given on page 144.

Exercise Programme for the First Six Weeks After the Birth (Normal Deliveries)

If you are breastfeeding, try to feed the baby before you do your exercises as your breasts will be more comfortable empty!

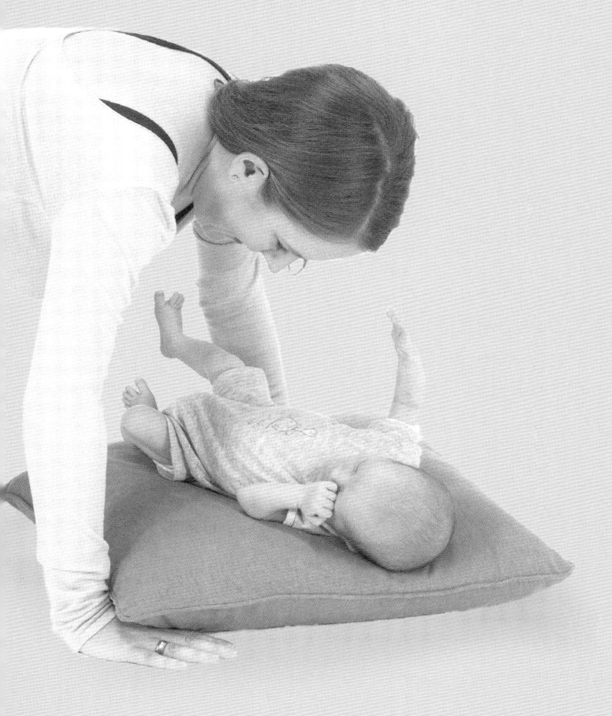

IMPORTANT NOTE

Arm exercises such as Arm Circles and Arm Openings may stimulate the flow of breast milk.

Start with:

Stabilizing on all Fours 50
The Pelvic Elevator (no longer going to the basement) 70
Pelvic Stability – Leg Slides, Knee Drops, Knee Folds 54–5
The Starfish 61
Shoulder Drops 66
Neck Rolls and Chin Tucks 62
The Pillow Squeeze 127
Baby Spine Curls with Pillow Squeeze 123
Big Squeeze 111
The Cat 155
The Star – Stage One (if you can lie on your front comfortably) 105
Ankle Circles 112
Demi Pliés in Turn Out 100
Walking on the Spot 124
The Dumb Waiter 101
Tennis Ball Rises 154

Then, when you are stronger add:

Sliding Down the Wall 135
The Corkscrew 125
Arm Circles Against the Wall 148
Arm Openings 137
Windows 132
The Oyster 149
Sitting Side Reach 86
Chest Expansion 131
The Diamond Press 107

Although swimming is a wonderful form of exercise, it is not recommended until after six weeks in case of infection.

Caesarean Births

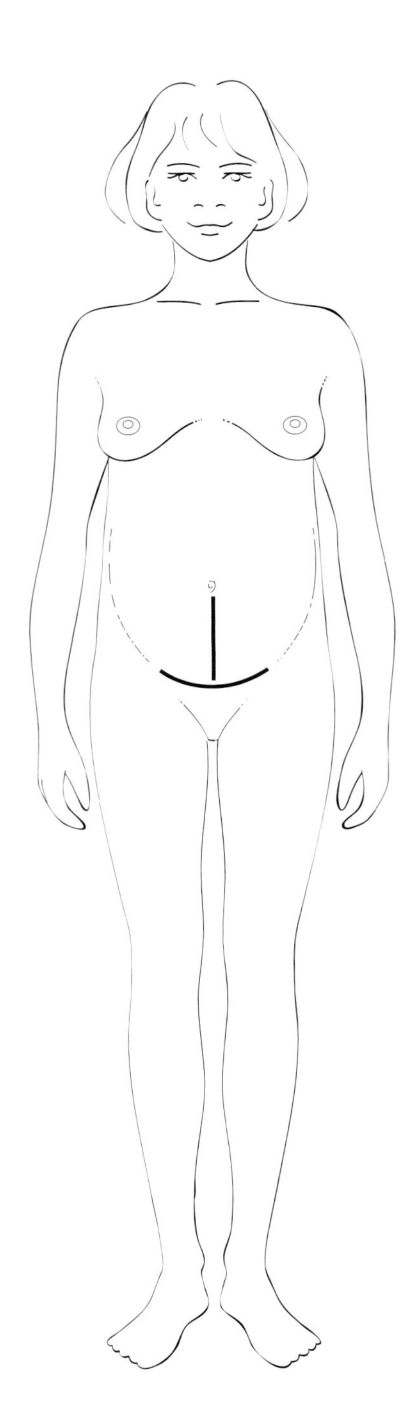

If you had a caesarean section, then you will find that for the first few days you will be uncomfortable because of the incision scar.

Moving about will be difficult. This is not surprising as you have had major abdominal surgery. Although your pelvic floor may be less traumatized by the birth, your baby has still been bouncing up and down on it for the last few weeks! You should start your pelvic floor exercises as soon as possible (ask your midwife or doctor what they recommend). The all-important transversus abdominis muscle will have been cut through during the operation. This does not mean that you cannot zip up and hollow, but it may feel a little strange to begin with. Persevere.

You may find yourself stooping because you are afraid of the pain and you are trying to protect the scar and stitches. This is a natural reaction but you should try to stand tall, remembering all the directions for Standing Well (page 16). Use your breathing to help you relax. You can gently support your abdomen with your hand and use your zip up and hollow to give you extra support.

Whenever you are getting on or off the bed, try to avoid awkward twisting movements or sitting up straight quickly. Someone should help you. Bend your knees and keep them together, then roll on to your side. Carefully push yourself up into sitting, allowing your legs to swing over the side of the bed and on to the floor. If the bed is at the right height, you can then stand up easily. If not, ask for the bed to be adjusted.

To get back into bed, sit on the edge of it as near to the head as possible. Zip up and hollow and lift your legs one at a time on to the bed. If necessary, lift your legs with your hands. Then, with the knees still bent, dig your heels into the mattress and lower yourself back towards the head of the bed with your hands.

When you have been given the go ahead to exercise you may start with the exercises below. You may need to wait a few days.

Circulation Exercises

If you have had a caesarean, your circulation will be affected so it is very important that you start to get the blood flowing again. At first you will have to practise these on the bed, but eventually you will be able to do them on the exercise mat.

Exercise 1
Sit tall on your bed with your legs stretched out in front of you hip-width apart and in parallel. Breathing normally but laterally, gently zip up and hollow and try to stay zipped as you point and flex your feet about 10 times. Pause, then do another 6 repetitions.

Exercise 2
Take your feet a little wider apart. Try to stay zipped and slowly and with control, circle your ankles 6 times in each direction.

Exercise 3
Lie on your bed in the Relaxation Position (page 26). Do slow Leg Slides as described on page 54. Repeat 6 times with each leg.

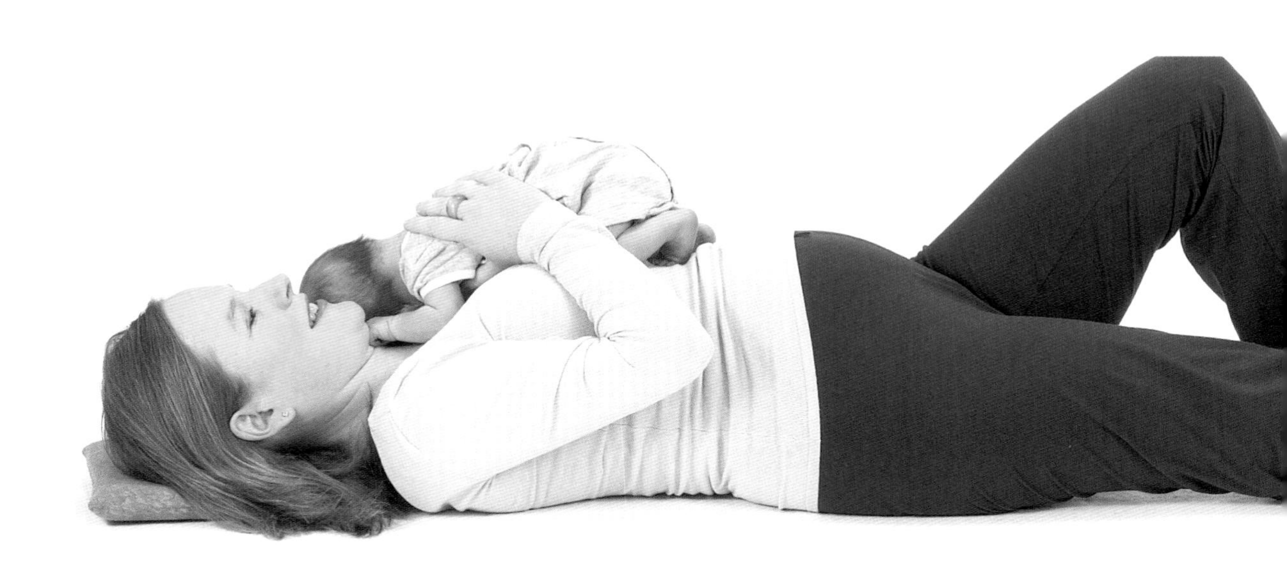

Breathing Exercise

If you had a general anaesthetic, then you should add the following exercise which will help to clear any secretions in the lungs left as a result of the anaesthetic. If they linger in the lungs you risk infection and for obvious reasons you will not be too keen on coughing at the moment, which would be the natural way to get rid of them.

Action

1. Sit tall in your bed or on a sturdy chair. The key is to lengthen up through the spine. You will find it hard to breathe with bad posture because your ribcage is closed down.
2. Place one hand on your scar to give it gentle support.
3. Breathe in wide and full and allow your ribs to expand; think of bucket handles lifting.
4. As you breathe out, focus on completely wringing out the lungs. Make a huffing noise to help and think of the bucket handles closing back down. Make sure you fully empty your lungs and relax the ribcage, allowing the breastbone to soften.
5. Repeat 8 times. Try to do this 5 times a day. Eventually you can add your zip up and hollow.

After a few weeks, when you are feeling stronger, and have been given the go ahead by your widwife or doctor, you can try the exercises listed below.

If you are breastfeeding, feed the baby before you do your exercises as your breasts will be more comfortable empty! Some arm exercises may stimulate the flow of breast milk.

Exercise Programme for the First Six Weeks After the Birth (Caesarean deliveries)

You *must* consult your doctor before you start exercising.

Start with:

Stabilizing on all Fours 50
The Pelvic Elevator (no longer going to the basement) 70
Pelvic Stability – Leg Slides and Knee Folds 54and 55
The Starfish 61
Shoulder Drops 66
Neck Rolls and Chin Tucks 62
Pillow Squeeze 127
The Cat 155
Ankle Circles 112
Demi Pliés in Turn Out 100
Walking on the Spot 124
The Dumb Waiter 101
Tennis Ball Rises 154

Then when you are stronger, add the following to your workout:

Baby Spine Curls with Pillow Squeeze 123
Sliding Down the Wall 135
The Corkscrew 125
Arm Circles Against the Wall 148
Windows 132
Chest Expansion 131
The Diamond Press 107
Big Squeeze 111

Although swimming is a wonderful form of exercise, it is not recommended until after six weeks in case of infection.

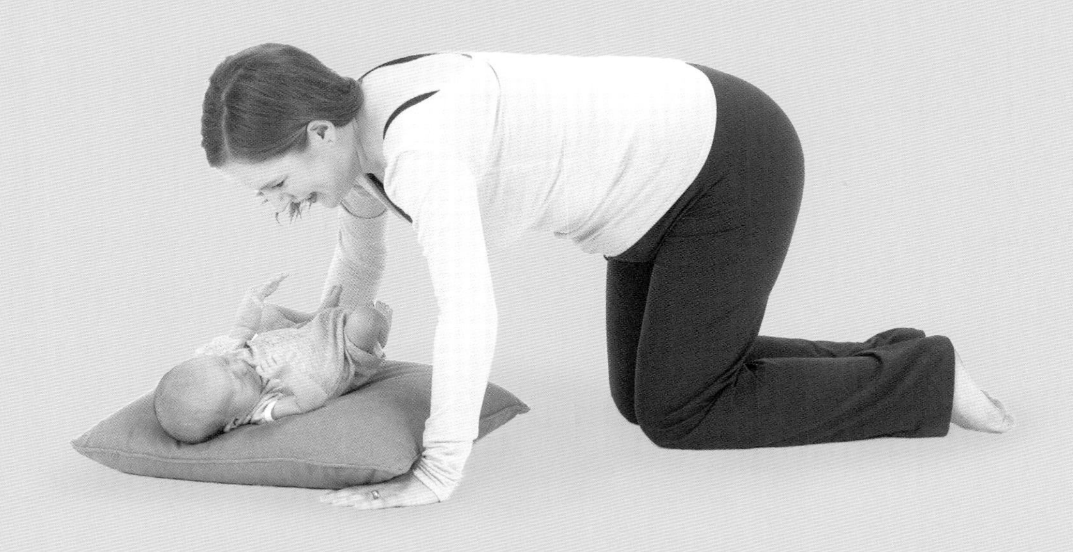

11 Getting Back Into Shape (Six Weeks Plus)

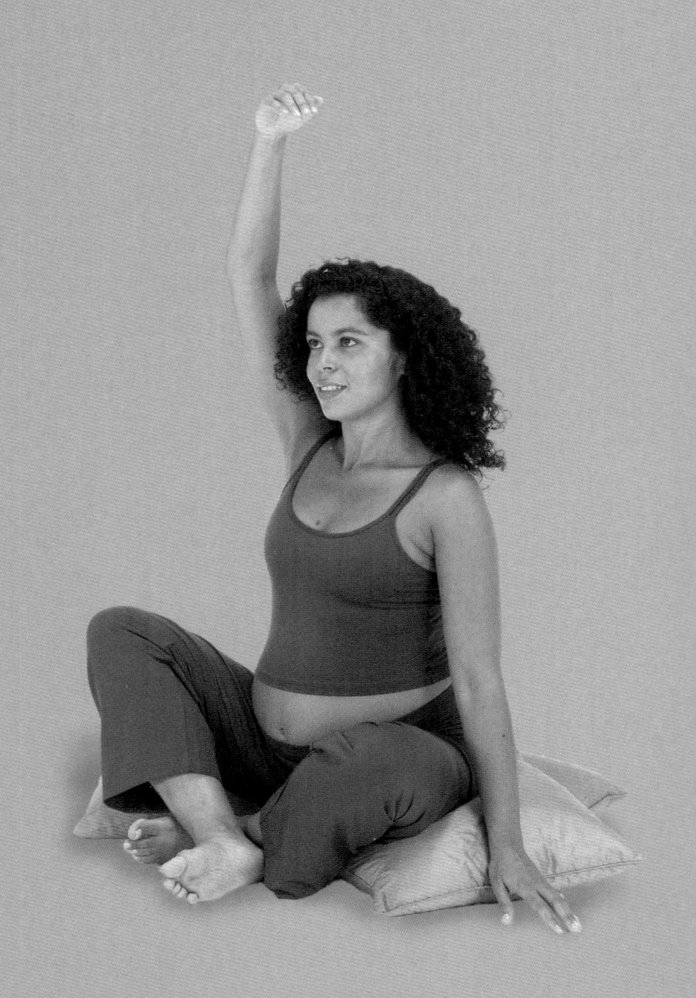

Normal Deliveries (Six Weeks Plus)

If you had a normal delivery and have had no complications after the birth, then after 6 weeks you can resume your normal exercise programme following the recommended guidelines given below. But it is worth bearing in mind that you are pregnant for 9 months and it takes 9 months to recover! It takes that long for your hormones to settle and for your body to return to normal. The key to getting your shape back quickly is to take things steadily and build up your strength gradually. After the 9-month period you can resume your pre-pregnant workouts.

The Six Weeks Plus programme draws on many of the exercises you have already learnt both before you were pregnant and during your pregnancy. The workouts have been designed to help give you the core strength you need to carry your baby and the essential baby paraphernalia that accompanies him or her wherever you go! You will be spending a lot of time bending over changing nappies, so you should include more extension work than before, which is much easier now you can lie on your stomach again! Exercises like the Diamond Press (page 107) and the Dart (page 91) feel wonderful because they move the spine the other way. If you find lying on your front uncomfortable for your breasts, buy some soft foam to put underneath. Be aware that sometimes a lot of arm work will stimulate milk flow. Keep your sessions short to avoid affecting your milk supply. Whether you are breastfeeding or bottle feeding, you will be spending a lot of time sitting nursing the baby, which is why we have included exercises like Arm Openings (page 137) to open out the chest and strengthen the mid-back muscles.

Hopefully by now your pelvic floor will be feeling more comfortable – the more pelvic floor work you can do, the better. The pelvic floor undergoes many changes in its connective tissue composition during the 6 weeks following the birth. It should gradually regain innervation of muscular groups lost during or prior to delivery. But the wide swings in your hormonal levels over the next few months will continue to affect connective tissue. As we have mentioned, if you had a difficult birth you may have suffered some nerve damage. You might find it helpful to give yourself some direct sensory feedback. Try inserting your finger into your vagina (perhaps in the bath) and then concentrate on squeezing your finger. Or perhaps more fun, during sex you can try squeezing your partner and asking if he can feel anything. Keep practising, but if there is no improvement check with your doctor. Sometimes extra medical help is needed to stimulate the muscles.

The hormonal changes which caused your ligaments to be lax in pregnancy, can continue to affect joint stability for up to 9 months after the birth. Therefore, as before, you should avoid wide ranges of movement, keep the limbs close to the body and movements smaller than normal, avoiding hamstring and adductor stretches or any exercise which puts pressure on the pubis symphysis, so all the guidelines given above apply.

In the chapter on the second trimester we explained diastasis recti where the abdominal wall separates as the uterus grows. This condition normally resolves itself spontaneously during the 6 weeks following the birth, but not always. In some cases the separation remains. The test for diastasis recti is commonly known as the 'rec' check. You can do it yourself, but it is best done by a professional (for example, your fitness instructor, midwife, health visitor, doctor or physiotherapist).

The 'Rec' Check

- Lie on your back with your knees bent and your feet flat on the floor.
- Place your fingers just above your navel and feel for two firm ridges of the rectus abdominis muscle. If you can feel a gap of more than two fingers you should continue with abdominal hollowing only and avoid any exercise that involves flexion (that is, a curl-up movement). See opposite for recommended exercises. Otherwise you can continue with the test.
- Breathe in, tuck your chin in gently and then as you breathe out, zip up and hollow and, sliding the free hand along the floor, gently curl up. Note what happens to the abdominals, then breathe in and curl back down.
- Hopefully, as you curled up, you will have felt the two sides of the abdominals firm and close together. If the gap remained at two fingers or more, or if you feel any bulging or doming, then you are not yet ready to do Curl Ups. If the gap closed to one finger and there is no doming, then you may start with gentle curl-up exercises.

Recommended Exercises for When You Still Have Diastasis Recti

If your abdominals are not ready for Curl Ups, don't worry. The more zipping up and hollowing you do the better. You can still exercise, working on the rest of your body. The pelvic stability exercises on pages 54 to 56 are an excellent way to strengthen the abdominals. Keep checking the rectus every week. Follow the workouts on pages 182–3 avoiding exercises marked with a star*.

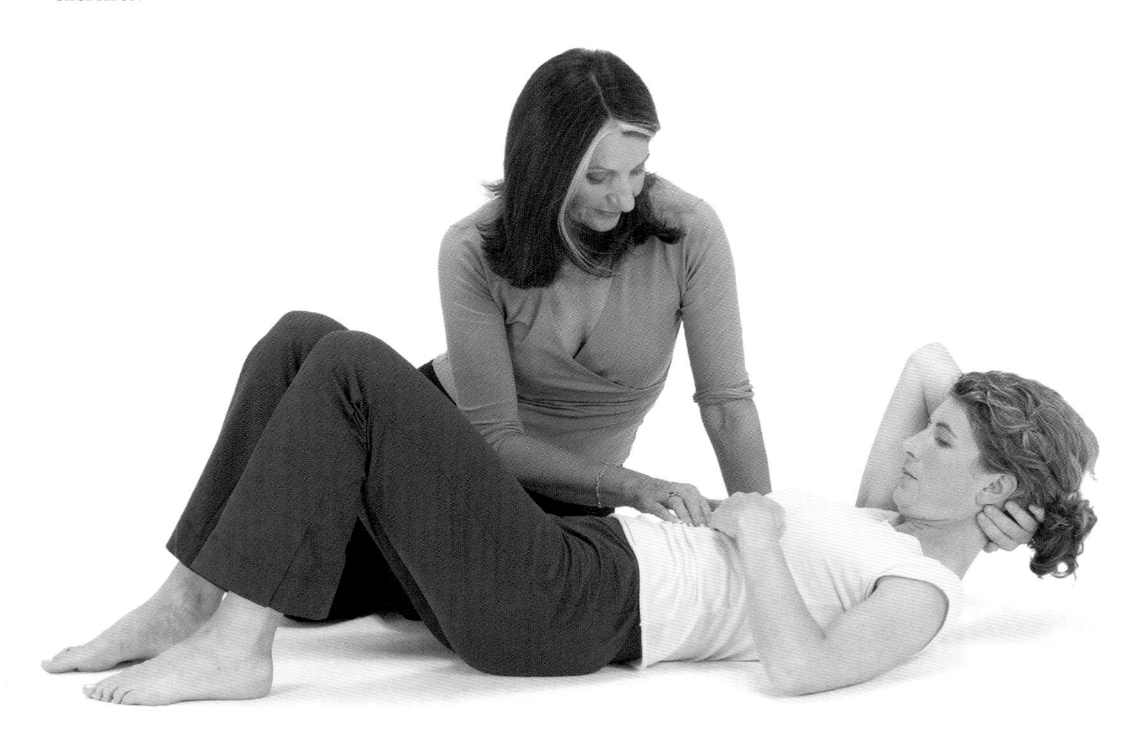

Caesarean Births (Six Weeks Plus)

If you had a caesarean birth you must remember that you have undergone major surgery. Once you have been given the go ahead by your practitioner you may begin a gentle exercise programme following the advice given on pages 174–6 and the exercise programme on page 177. However, because of the incision you should avoid any curl-up action (flexion) for at least 5 months. You should also be cautious with any exercise that requires a lot of abdominal strength. Don't despair, the simple action of zipping and hollowing will help you to strengthen your abdominals and regain your figure. Follow the recommended workouts given but leave out any exercise with a curl-up action. Continue to do your pelvic floor exercises, bearing in mind that although this area avoided the trauma of vaginal delivery, it will still have been weakened during the latter stages of pregnancy as it bore the additional weight of the uterus and baby.

Body Control Pilates has helped me through all three of my pregnancies. I was doing Pilates right up to the birth of all three babies. It helped enormously with my back problems. I discovered stomach muscles I never knew I had and these strong muscles have really helped me get back into shape. Now ten years on I have a better figure than before.

– *Lucinda Fraser*

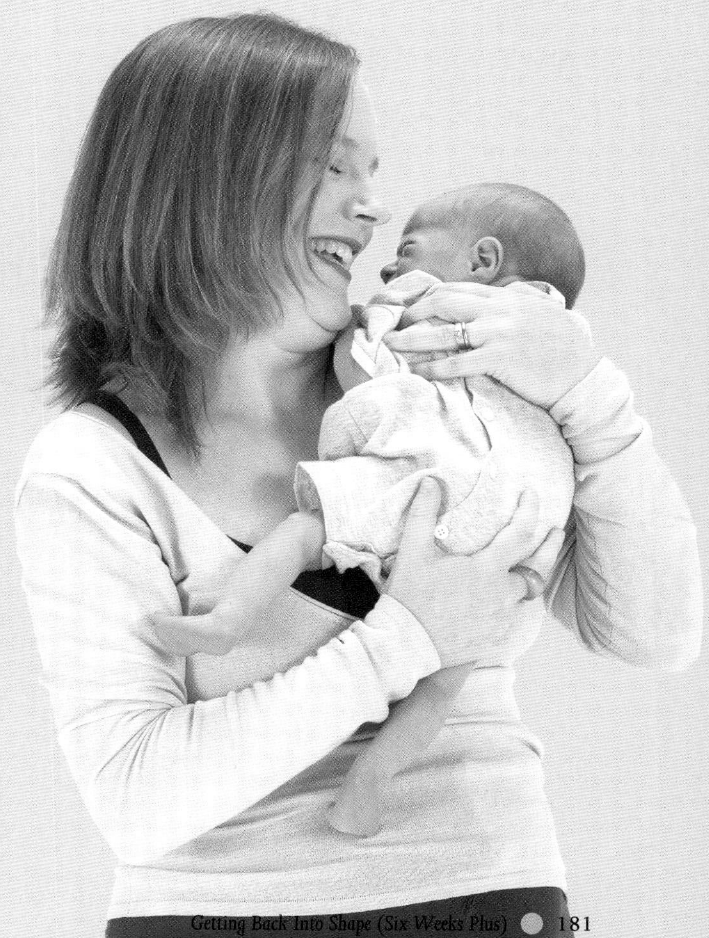

Getting Back Into Shape Workouts (after 6 weeks)

The following workouts should not be started until at least 6 weeks after the birth and then only when your midwife/doctor gives you the go-ahead. Mothers who have had a caesarean delivery or who still have diastasis recti (see pages 180–1) should avoid all exercises marked with a star*.

If you are breastfeeding, try to feed the baby before you do your exercises as your breasts will be more comfortable empty!

Take time with the transition from one exercise to the next – roll on to your side.

How soon you return to your pre-pregnant workouts will depend on your individual level of fitness. It is very hard to give general guidelines on this but you should remember that your hormones will take up to 9 months to return to normal, which means your joints may still be unstable. Build your strength gradually. If you have been exercising throughout your pregnancy you will have laid the best possible foundations to getting your figure back. Be patient and listen to your body.

Workout One

Monkey Bends with Arms 129
Tennis Ball Rises 154
The Corkscrew 125
Sitting Side Reach 86
Baby Spine Curls with Pillow Squeeze 123
*Curl Ups 68
*Hip Rolls (Level One only) 81
*Single Leg Stretch (Level One only) 75
Arm Openings 137
Pelvic Floor Exercises: Elevator, Figure of Eight, Emergency Stop 70, 171, 172
Arm Circles Against the Wall 148
Single Leg Circles 102
The Diamond Press 107
The Big Squeeze 111
The Cat 155
The Rest Position 93

Workout Two

Baby Spine Curls with Pillow Squeeze 123
*Curl Ups 68
Chalk Circles 151
The Hundred (breathing only) 78
Pelvic Stability Check 150
Windows 132
The Pelvic Elevator and The Emergency Stop 70 and 71
Threading a Needle 110
The Dart 91
The Rest Position 93
Abductor and Adductor Lifts (no weights) 87 and 89
Rolling Down a Wall 84
The Dumb Waiter 101
Arm Circles Against the Wall 148
The Scapular Squeeze 160
The Pillow Squeeze 127

Workout Three

The Full Starfish 65
Shoulder Drops 66
Neck Rolls and Chin Tucks 62
*Curl Ups 68
*Hip Rolls (Level One only) 81
Pelvic Stability Check 150
The Star 105
The Diamond Press 107
The Cat 155
The Rest Position 93
Side-lying Circles 134
Sitting Side Reach 86
Rolling Down a Wall 84
Walking on the Spot 124
Pole Raises 152
The Pelvic Elevator and Figure of Eight 70 and 171
Baby Spine Curls with Pillow Squeeze 123
Hip Flexor Stretch 72

Workout Four

Demi Pliés in Turn Out 100
The Corkscrew 125
Standing Tarzan 157
Back Press 158
Baby Spine Curls with Pillow Squeeze 123
Single Leg Circles 102
*Curl Ups 68
*Single Leg Stretch (Level One only) 75
Ankle Circles 112
Windows 132
*Hip Rolls (Level One only) 81
The Oyster 149
The Big Squeeze 111
The Diamond Press 107
Treading a Needle 110
The Rest Position 93
The Pelvic Elevator and The Emergency Stop
70 and 71
Arm Openings 137

Workout Five

Pelvic Stability Check 150
Shoulder Drops 66
*Curl Ups 68
The Hundred (breathing only) 78
Arm Circles Against the Wall 148
The Cat 155
The Dart 91
The Rest Position 93
Rolling Down a Wall 84
The Scapular Squeeze 160
Pole Raises 152
Bow and Arrow 126
The Pelvic Elevator, Figure of Eight, Emergency Stop
70, 171, 71
The Star 105
Threading a Needle 110
Side-lying Circles 134
The Full Starfish 65
Chalk Circles 151

Bibliography

James F. Clapp, *Exercising Through Your Pregnancy*, Addicus, 2002

Sheila Kitzinger, *The New Pregnancy and Childbirth*, Penguin, 1997

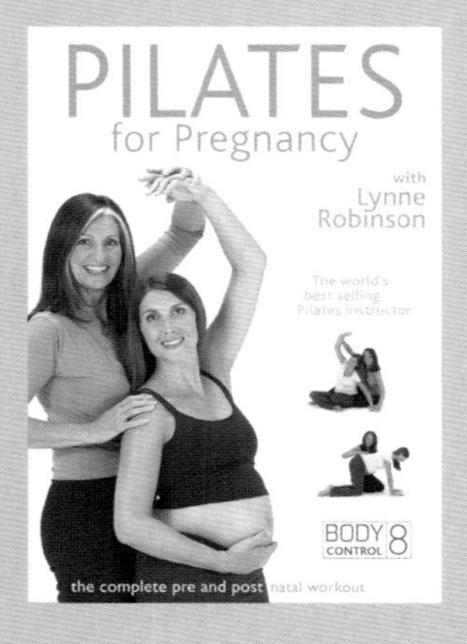

Pilates for Pregnancy Video and DVD
© Firefly Entertainment 2004
Available from all good video/DVD stockists
DVD £14.99
VHS £10.99

Watch out for new titles!

Other Body Control Pilates books

BODY CONTROL THE PILATES WAY
0 330 36945 8 / £7.99

THE MIND–BODY WORKOUT
0 330 36946 6 / £12.99

PILATES THE WAY FORWARD
0 330 37081 2 / £12.99

THE OFFICIAL BODY CONTROL PILATES MANUAL
0 330 39327 8 / £12.99

PILATES GYM
0 330 48309 9 / £12.99

THE BODY CONTROL PILATES BACK BOOK
0 330 48311 0 / £9.99

THE BODY CONTROL PILATES
POCKET TRAVELLER
0 330 49106 7 / £4.99

INTELLIGENT EXERCISE WITH PILATES & YOGA
0 333 98952 X / £16.99

THE PERFECT BODY THE PILATES WAY
0 330 48953 4 / £12.99

PILATES PLUS DIET
0 330 48954 2 / £10.99

THE COMPLETE CLASSIC PILATES METHOD
1 4050 0558 0 / £18.99

These are available from all good bookshops,
or can be ordered direct from:
Book Services By Post
PO Box 29
Douglas
Isle of Man IM99 IBQ

Credit card hotline +44 (0) 1624 675 137
Postage and packing free in the UK

Further Information

Pilates

For general information on the Body Control Pilates Method; to find a qualified teacher; for information on how to become a teacher; and for details on books, videos and other products, please visit the Body Control Pilates website at www.bodycontrol.co.uk
or write to:

The Body Control Pilates Association
6, Langley Street,
London, WC2H 9JA,
England.

Pilates During Pregnancy Programmes are available at:

The Body Control Pilates Studio
David Lloyd Club
Point West,
116 Cromwell Road,
London SW7 4XR
Telephone: 020 7244 8060

Pregnancy

For general information and advice:

The National Childbirth Trust –
Alexandra House,
Oldham Terrace,
London W3 6NH
Central office:
Telephone: 0870 444 8707
Website: www.nctpregnancyandbabycare.com

Specialist Furniture

Advance Seating Design
Unit H, Fieldway,
Metropolitan Park, Greenford
Middlesex UB6 8UN
Telephone: 020 8578 4308
Website: www.asd.co.uk

The Belly bag
www.p4pilates.com

Acknowledgements

Writing this book has been both a huge responsibility and an amazing source of joy. Very similar in fact to the feelings I have when teaching Pilates to a pregnant client. I am always excited and have a sense of being very privileged, but at the same time conscious that I have double the responsibility to give good direction and advice – there are two persons present in class! I have been lucky enough, and honoured, to teach many pregnant clients, some of them until just hours before they gave birth. I have seen how Pilates has helped them enjoy their pregnancies, free from many of the commonly associated aches and pains. Nothing beats the moment when they bring the baby into class.

My first thank you is therefore to those clients who trusted me with their bodies at this very special time.

Then I have many colleagues to thank. It is always fun to work with Jackie Knox. She has a great reputation as a talented and knowledgeable physiotherapist yet seems to be able to make even the most complicated anatomical discussion lively and interesting. We have worked closely together to create a very popular pregnancy course for our Body Control Pilates teachers. Many of those teachers were anxious to know which exercises were safe, which were beneficial. Much of this book was derived from their questions and experiences. Thank you, Jackie, for sharing your wisdom with us.

A big thank you to the lovely Philippa Satchwell, who teaches on our course and who very kindly read through the manuscript and advised us on many points. Philippa's neighbour, Lisa, is a midwife and she was also gracious enough to check the script to see if it fitted in with current midwifery ideas. Thank you, Lisa.

You will see the stunningly beautiful pregnant ladies who agreed to be photographed for this book. Don't they look amazing? You would never guess that the shoot took place on the three hottest days on record. Their stamina and patience was incredible. Sharon, Emma and Claudine you are real stars! Congratulations on your lovely babies. Thank you also Wilf and mum Catriona.

Sadly, this was the last project on which I worked with publisher Gordon Wise; I hope he is happy with the finished project and I wish him every success in his new job, although I miss him terribly. However, Ingrid, Jacqui, Rafi and Liz are all looking after me very well.

And lastly, a personal note. The research for the book brought back many memories of my own pregnancies: the backache, swollen ankles and heartburn – I wish I had known about Pilates then – but the aches and pains were well worth it. Now my two gorgeous daughters Rebecca and Emily are in their early twenties and university graduates. Thank you girls for putting up with your 'crazy' mother – I am incredibly proud of you both.

Lynne Robinson